WEIGHTS
for
50+

WEIGHTS

for

50+

Building Strength, Staying Healthy and Enjoying an Active Lifestyle

DR. KARL KNOPF

photography by Robert Holmes

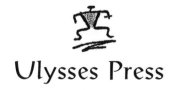

Ulysses Press

Published in the United States by
Ulysses Press
P.O. Box 3440
Berkeley, CA 94703
www.ulyssespress.com

ISBN 1-56975-511-6
Library of Congress Control Number 2005930013

Printed in Canada by Transcontinental Printing

10 9 8 7 6 5 4 3 2 1

Editorial/Production	Ashley Chase, Lily Chou, Claire Chun, Nicholas Denton-Brown, Matt Orendorff, Steven Zah Schwartz
Cover design	Leslie Henriques
Photography	Robert Holmes
Models	Karl Knopf, Toni Silver, Grant Bennett, Vivian Gunderson, Phyllis Ritchie, Michael O'Meara

Distributed by Publishers Group West

Please Note
This book has been written and published strictly for informational purposes, and in no way
should be used as a substitute for consultation with health care professionals. You should not
consider educational material herein to be the practice of medicine or to replace consultation
with a physician or other medical practitioner. The author and publisher are providing you
with information in this work so that you can have the knowledge and can choose, at your
own risk, to act on that knowledge. The author and publisher also urge all readers to be
aware of their health status and to consult health care professionals before beginning any
health program.

contents

part one:

getting
started

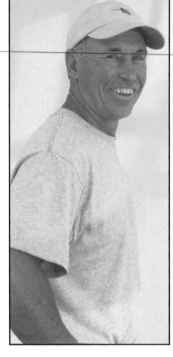

grow strong, not old

Many people let their age exclude them from being the healthiest and fittest person they can be. Everyday we have the ability to determine how we want to age. To a large extent how well we age has to do with how we eat, sleep, think and move. Our attitude towards aging largely influences how we age. If you view the process as a time of decline and frailty, you will be fighting each birthday rather than making every year the best year of your life. Also, if you allow advertisers to make you feel bad about living, then you will continue to deny aging rather than embrace it.

One of my favorite 90-plus students told me she loves aging, especially when you consider the alternative. A dynamic 100-year-old woman in my class said that the best part of hitting the century mark is that there is less peer pressure. When asked whether she cares about her wrinkles, she said, "Heck no! I have earned every one of them." Another student once told me, "Age is just a number and mine is not listed." A 75-year-old student told me that she didn't care about her age because she feels better and more empowered than ever before. She went on to say that how you feel and act is more important than the numbers of candles on a cake and that being active everyday makes her feel better than the day before.

The people who live long and thrive often report that the success of their aging was largely influenced by their positive attitude, being physically active, eating healthily, moderating their consumption of alcohol, avoiding cigarettes, getting adequate rest and sleep and staying socially engaged. If we want society to change its attitude about aging, we need to start bragging about our age rather than denying it. We also need to be proactive and take steps today to positively influence our health.

More and more research supports the conclusion that we can control our own aging.

Many scientists believe that with a healthy lifestyle, we may be able to turn back the biological clock 10 to 20 years or at least slow it down. A healthy active person ages approximately half a percent a year, compared to an inactive person with poor health habits, who ages at approximately two percent a year. If you do the math, you can see how a healthy lifestyle can make a significant difference over a period of a lifetime. Fortunately for all of us, the fountain of youth has been discovered. It is not found in a bottle or in a pill or even in an injection. It is found in a daily dose of prudent exercise that includes strength training.

As we grow older, we expect certain changes to occur. We may notice that we gain weight, have less energy and are not as strong as we once were and have less muscle tone. Aging is not to blame! Most of the time the blame falls squarely on an inactive lifestyle. Regular exercise is the single most important thing we can do to retard the effects of aging. How we age has little to do with our chronological age but rather our physiological age. What we do today plays a significant role in how we will age tomorrow.

In the end we can not become what we need to be by remaining what we are.

—Max De Pree

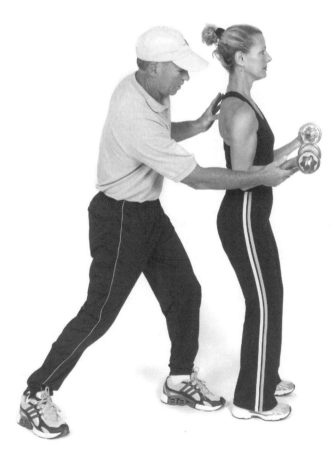

Author Karl Knopf makes some adjustments.

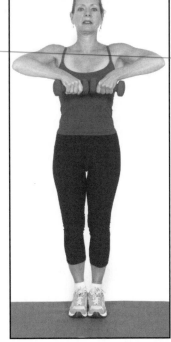

fit for life

Hippocrates said it so well more than 2000 years ago: "All parts of the body, which have function, if used in moderation and exercised to which each is accustomed, become thereby healthy and well developed and age slowly. But if left idle become liable to disease, defective in growth and age quickly." Mickey Mantle said the same thing, but in a simpler way: "If I knew I was going to live this long I would have taken better care of myself."

Strength training is the single most critical step you can take to retard aging. The human body has over 400 voluntary muscles—it's a machine that was designed for movement. Yet, in this technology-driven age, we consistently invest in products that reduce our need to move. Do you remember the days when you had to get out of the car to open the garage door? Or get up to change the TV channel? Even these simple bouts of physical activity required muscular strength. Unfortunately, all these wonderful labor-saving devices that we use daily hasten the process of *sarcopenia* (age-related loss of muscle mass and strength). To keep our muscles from withering away from disuse, we must challenge them frequently.

Young people frequently exercise to look better. In middle age, people often exercise for the health of it. However, in order to age well and remain fully independent, we need to exercise for the function of it. Too often, older people find that many of the activities of daily living that they once found simple have become challenging. Many of my older students joined my classes because steps seemed higher than they used to be, chairs were harder to get out of, and even the act of lifting a bag of groceries caused strain. Much of the decline often associated with normal aging has more to do with a loss of muscular strength and function than the number of trips around the sun.

A great deal of strength is lost between the ages of 30 and 50. If a person participates in a regular strength-training routine, the loss of strength can be minimized. Fortunately, it is never too late to turn your fitness life around. Numerous studies have proven that both men and women in their 80s and 90s can regain their strength and function by engaging in sensible and regular strength training; in cases of arthritis, several studies have shown that when the muscles around an arthritic joint get stronger, the load placed on that joint decreases. I have personally witnessed a woman in my strength class lose about 30 pounds and dramatically improve her ability to get around; she no longer uses a walker and can pick things up off the floor easily, which she was unable to do a year ago. Today she has more energy and is having a lot more fun than she ever remembered. All these positive results can be derived by a slight reduction in calories to lose weight slowly and permanently, combined with a daily dose of strength training and aerobic exercise.

If You Rest, You Rust

People who do not engage in a regular strength-training routine throughout their lives will lose 40 to 50 percent of their muscle mass and 50 percent of their muscular strength by age 65. This loss is not without consequence—these people can become so weak that doing simple daily activities becomes very difficult. A recent study revealed just how much negative impact a sedentary lifestyle can have on aging. The study looked at adults aged 55 to 64 and found that 40 percent of women had a difficult time lifting and carrying 10 pounds; 20 percent of men within this age bracket found the same task difficult. This study also revealed that almost 25 percent of both men and women had a difficult time walking a quarter of a mile briskly. The saddest part of this report stated that

by age 65, untrained individuals had lost as much as 80 percent of their strength.

The chart below gives you an idea of the percent of muscle loss in some major muscle groups.

Muscle group	percentage of strength loss
Back & arms	30–40%
Legs	47%
Hand & grip strength	42%

This decline can be responsible for loss of independent living skills and can exacerbate existing disabilities. While this information is both alarming and discouraging, the good news is that it is never too late to feel great and recapture some of the strength and stamina we had in our younger days. All it takes is a sensible and regular dose of strength training to prevent sarcopenia.

Benefits of Strength Training

Although there are numerous benefits that arise from strength training, perhaps the most obvious benefit is maintaining existing strength. Doctors Bortz and Nelson, experts in the field of older adult wellness, agree that the best way to stay out of a nursing home and maintain or regain independence is to keep legs strong.

Recent information suggests that strength training once a

week is all we need to do to maintain strength. Strength training three times a week provides optimal results. However, performing strength training twice a week yields 80 percent of the benefits that you gain from working out three times a week.

In addition to maintaining existing strength, we can also increase muscle mass and regain lost muscle with regular strength training. Improvements in muscular strength and endurance make everyday tasks, such as opening jars and getting up from the floor, easier. Don't become too concerned with looking like a body builder, though. Most women and people over the age of 50 lack the amount of testosterone needed to develop large muscles.

Strength training also retards aging. One study asked college-age students to identify which older adults, all belonging to the same age group, looked most youthful: those who strength-trained, those who swam, or those who ran. The overwhelming response was that those who lifted weights looked the youngest.

Strength training, when combined with sensible eating habits and moderate aerobic exercise, facilitates weight loss, decreases body fat and helps keep weight off. Muscles are a furnace that burns calories.

Some experts suggest that one pound of fat burns only 3 to 5 calories a day whereas a pound of muscle burns 35 to 50 calories a day. Thus, the more muscle mass we have, the more calories we will burn while at work or rest. People who have a higher percent of muscle mass have a higher resting metabolic rate than sedentary individuals and thus are burning more calories.

Here are some additional benefits derived from strength training.

Decreases arthritic and lower back pain. Muscles provide structure around the joint, creating an internal brace to support and also lessen the load on the joint.

Increases bone density. When strength training, the muscle pulls on the bone, requiring the bone to remodel itself to get stronger and provide a more solid base of support. The integrity of the bone is directly related to the forces applied to it. If a person lives a zoolike existence, their fragile bones will break easily against the slightest force.

Improves glucose tolerance and insulin sensitivity. Diabetes is increasing in the United States at alarming rates. The physical activity that strength training provides improves the way the body utilizes sugar and will lessen the risk of developing diabetes.

Improves mobility and functional ability. Maintaining or regaining strength allows us to do what we want to do, when we want to do it.

Improves balance and prevents falls. Having adequate leg strength allows us to catch ourselves when we trip, preventing a fall and perhaps a broken bone. Strength training also increases bone density so that the bones can withstand the impact of a fall better. In addition, it will be easier to get up if we do fall.

Improves posture and self-image. Strength training correctly can reverse the Dowagers hump and other outward manifestations of poor posture. Proper strength training can assist us in regaining an upright youthful appearance.

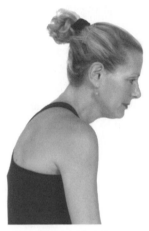

Dowagers hump

Combats depression. Studies have found that older people who strength-trained for ten weeks had reductions in depression and improvements in self-esteem. This suggests that strength training gives a sense of empowerment and the idea that it is never too late to improve.

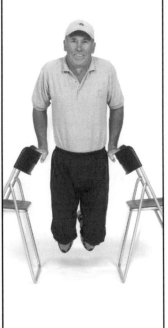

what is strength training?

According to the National Strength and Conditioning Association, strength training is defined as the use of progressive resistance methods to increase one's ability to exert force or resist a force. Basically, strength training is challenging your muscles in a sensible and progressive manner.

It is critical to use muscles in the manner they were designed to be used; unused muscles will no longer work efficiently. Use it or lose it has real meaning for older adults. In strength training, it is not where you start that is important but where you end up. I have had numerous students start my class unable to get out of a chair without the use of their hands, but after performing some of the exercises in this book, they can now sit down and get up from a chair with ease, walk around the mall all day or even get down on the floor and play with the grandkids.

Different Types

Strength training can take many forms, from lifting your own body against the resistance of gravity to using weights or exercise bands to challenge your muscles. Many people confuse the terms *weight lifting, weight training, strength training* and *progressive resistance exercise.*

Weight lifting is a competitive form of strength training using Olympic-style lifts such as the "snatch" and the "clean and jerk."

Weight training is the process of lifting weights, whether they are dumbbells, barbells or weight machines.

Strength training is the application of resistance to movement to increase one's ability to exert force. The muscle does not know nor care what is providing the resistance, so engaging in a method that you enjoy is the key to success. This can include the use of anything from weights to exercise bands to even the resistance of the water.

Progressive resistance exercise is when a person progressively overloads the muscles (by making the load and movement more difficult) by adding more resistance as the move gets easier. The load

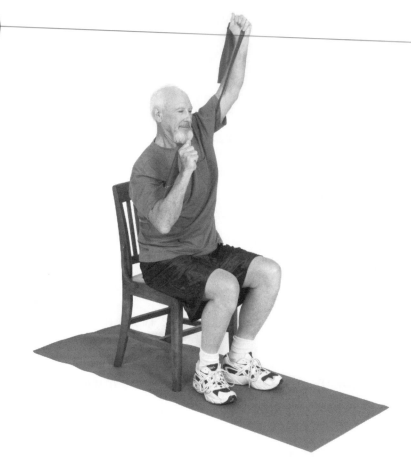

mass and muscular endurance. The most common technique is *isotonic progressive resistance exercise*. The other methods are called *isometric* and *isokinetic progressive resistance exercise.*

Isotonic Progressive Resistance Exercise

Isotonic progressive resistance exercise is the most traditional method of strength training, generally using free weights, barbells or machines that utilize stacked weights or even exercise bands; isotonic progressive resistance is the style this book predominately uses. Isotonic exercise is convenient; the down side, however, is that it does not accommodate to changes in strength at different angles. Muscles can be stronger or weaker depending on the angle engaged. As the muscle contracts along the range of motion, the angle of the joint affects the strength at that angle.

To test the concept of your muscle's strength being dependent on the angle used, try placing a heavy jug of milk in each hand with your arms alongside your body. Now try to curl your hands towards your shoulders. Did you notice that at certain points/angles the milk jug seemed heavier than at other angles? The weight did not change but the angle made the weight feel heavier at certain points.

can be applied several ways: with weights, exercise tubing or, in water, hand paddles.

The following is a cute example of progressive resistance exercise:

Begin by standing in a comfortable position with plenty of room to move. With a 5-pound potato sack in each hand, lift your arms out to the sides 10 times. When that gets easy, grab a 25-pound potato sack in each hand and lift your arms 10 times. Once that becomes easy, start placing potatoes in the sack. Or another method is to buy a Great Dane puppy and then lift it every day. As the puppy gains weight, your muscles will get progressively stronger to adapt to the new heavier load.

While that was meant to be humorous, it does represent the theory behind progressive resistance exercise: Start at a comfortable load and slowly try to complete more reps each time, adding more load as your muscles get stronger and the movement gets easier.

Several methods are available to develop strength, muscle

Isotonic moves are involved in most of our daily activities, from lifting a bag of groceries to picking up a grandchild.

Isokinetic Exercise

In isokinetic exercise, you contract the muscle through the full range of motion against a resistance lever at a prescribed speed and load. Generally, isokinetic exercise machines are more expensive than isotonic machines and devices.

Isometric Exercise

Isometric exercise involves exerting muscular force against an immovable object, creating a static contraction. This method is often used with extremely weak individuals and with people with ailments such as arthritis, where movement of the joint is not desired. This type of training will not significantly develop muscle size or muscular endurance but will develop strength at the joint angle in which the exercise is performed. The advantage of isometric exercise is that it does not require equipment. The disadvantages are: it can raise blood pressure to dangerous levels; the strength gain is specific to the angle the move is performed; there is little transfer of strength to functional skills or sports.

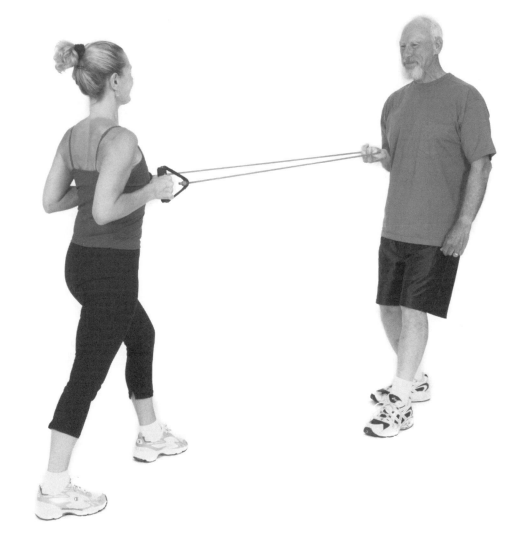

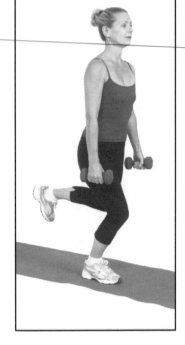

your program

Any successful exercise program should be fun, improve function, and assist you in becoming more physically fit and independent. A well-designed strength-training program can address each of these elements, but be aware that strength training can be done incorrectly. When designing a strength-training routine, it is critical that you use the correct dose to get the ideal response.

The first step in designing a safe and sane program is to cater to your health status and personal goals. Pay special attention to your problem areas and do what you feel is best for you. The areas that are at most risk of injury are the neck area, the lower back, the knees and the shoulders. These areas need to be trained, not strained.

Since so much misinformation abounds about strength training, it is important to use scientifically proven information rather than anecdotal information. Listen to your body and heed what it says. When in doubt, consult your health professional. In fact, it is always wise to inform your

health professional before you start any exercise program. However, if you start slow and don't strain, most health professionals will be very supportive of you engaging in a sensible strength-training routine. If you have health issues such as arthritis, heart and blood pressure issues, or bone density concerns, it would be smart to have your health professional review your program before starting.

As you design your program, ask yourself the following questions:

- What is the goal of my strength-training program?
- Do I have joint or other health problems that need special consideration?

- Will my program assist me to function more freely?
- Does my routine address all the major muscle groups of my body?
- Am I addressing only the surface muscles and neglecting the stabilizer muscles and core muscles of the body?
- If I feel worse after working out, am I doing more than I'm ready for or am I doing exercises that don't match my health?

Every exercise program should be customized for your unique characteristics. When evaluating an exercise, see if your exercise passes the following Benefits to Risk Ratio Test.

<table>
<tr><td colspan="2">SAMPLE ROUTINE</td></tr>
</table>

A sample routine may look something like this:	
Warm up	5–10 minutes
Aerobic activity	20–30 minutes*
Strength training	20–30 minutes*
Cool down and stretching	5–10 minutes

* The order of aerobic activity and strength training can be switched.

- Why am I doing this exercise?
- What are the benefits of this exercise?
- What are the risks of this exercise and can it be modified to make it safer?
- How do I feel while doing this exercise?
- How do I feel after doing this exercise?
- Could I receive the same benefits from doing a different exercise?
- Bonus: Does my doctor and/or therapist support this exercise?

If the exercise fails the above criteria, look for another exercise. There is no perfect exercise.

The Routine

A proper exercise program should include a warm-up period to prepare the body for exercise. The older the human machine, the longer and more therapeutic the warm-up should be. A warm-up can take several forms. It can consist of light aerobic activity that limbers up the muscles you plan to engage. It can also be a very light version of the exercise you plan to perform. The best method is to combine the two, doing a few minutes of aerobic exercise to warm up the body and then a light set of each exercise before you do your more formal sets.

The rest of the program should include cardiovascular training, often referred to as "cardio" or aerobics, and then perform muscular strength and endurance training. After the workout, a cool-down period is prudent. This allows your body to taper off from your workout. You do not want to stop abruptly. It is recommended that you walk around slowly then find a place to spend 5–15 minutes stretching the muscles you engaged in your workout. I've included some safe and effective stretches in this book; you may also want to check out my other book, *Stretching for 50+*, for a wider range of stretches.

Cross-training is a good way to avoid injury. An example of cross-training is strength training on Monday, Wednesday and Friday, swimming on Tuesday and Thursday, taking a walk on Saturday and resting on Sunday. Also, it is okay to break the aerobic exercise into three 10-minute bouts throughout the day. Cross-training does not mean combining aerobic training with strength training by carrying weights while walking or jogging, for instance. While this may sound like a great way to multi-task, it is only inviting orthopedic injuries. Wearing ankle weights on the ankles while walking is often implicated in hip and knee problems.

An important concept to keep in mind is not to become complacent about your exercise program. Be mindful of your body mechanics at all times. In other words, pay attention to what you are doing. When strength training, it is important that you control the weight and not let the weight control you. About every three to four months, you should change your workout around a bit so that you don't get bored and your body doesn't get accustomed to the work it's performing.

Pre- and Post-Strength Training

Always start with a 5- to 10-minute warm-up of the body before lifting weights. Stretch after your workout.

If you find your muscles are very sore after exercising, you are trying to do too much too soon. Muscle soreness results when you cause minor trauma to your muscles and connective tissue by asking them to do more than they are ready to perform. If you start and progress slowly and listen to your body, you should be able to avoid what is called "delayed muscle soreness," or next-day soreness. To avoid muscle soreness, always warm up then stretch, and then exercise carefully and again stretch at the end of your workout. Remember the two-hour rule: If you are sore two hours post-exercise, then you overworked and need to back off to an intensity that does not cause discomfort. The phrase "no pain, no gain" is insane.

Selecting Weight Load

Beginners should choose an amount that enables them to do at least one set of 12 reps; follow this procedure for one to two weeks. After two weeks, add a second set. It is best to do one set then rest for 45 seconds, then do a second set of the same exercise. When you can do two sets of 12 reps without straining, it is time to add just enough resistance so that it is difficult to do 6–8 reps; from here, work yourself back up to 12–15 reps. Add resistance in small increments

Two ways to improve strength is by adding more load or adding more reps. The more fit/active the person is when he or she starts, the slower his or her gains will be when compared to a beginner. Remember, you are only competing against yourself.

Deciding Reps and Sets

Each workout should not exceed 12 exercises and should engage the major muscles of the body.

Each set should consist of 8–15 repetitions. The more reps you perform, the more focus you place on muscular endurance. Choosing lower reps emphasizes strength and power. Most experts suggest that older adults should find a load that can be done comfortably 6–8 times, gradually increasing the reps until they can do 15 reps with good form before they increase the resistance and then start the sequence all over again. Try to do at least 2–3 sets of each exercise.

Frequency

The key to a successful strength-training program is to start slow and progress in a sensible manner. Try to strength train a minimum of two days a week; three times a week would be ideal. Over-training can occur when you are doing too much, working out too often and not allowing your body adequate time to rest and repair itself. This often occurs in newcom-

ers who try to do too many sets with too many reps at a pace that is too fast. To avoid this: Train, don't strain!

Training Progressions and Plateaus

Training progression should not exceed 5 to 10 percent a week. In the beginning, your strength increases quickly as you learn how to coordinate

---

COMMON TERMS

Atrophy: a decrease in muscle size as a result of inactivity

Circuit training: a series of different exercises done with no significant rest in between each set

Contraction: muscles utilizing energy and expending heat to exert a force

Concentric contraction: an isotonic contraction in which muscle length shortens, e.g., bringing a glass of water to your mouth

Eccentric movement: a movement in which the muscle lengthens while resisting the load, e.g., bringing down the glass of water slowly from your mouth.

Extension: making the joint angle larger

Flexion: making the joint angle smaller

Rep (or Repetition): the number of times you perform a movement

Set: a grouping of repetitions

the equipment. A beginner can expect to see gains in strength, size and firmness after six to eight weeks. However, at some point improvement will slow down and then stop. Plateaus in strength often occur after the first few months of training. Don't get discouraged—just realize that improvements will take longer and will not be as noticeable.

As long as you are not feeling bad, good things are still going on inside the muscle. When you reach a plateau, it is time to tweak your routine by changing the exercises or changing the number of reps and/or sets. Athletes who reach a plateau may even take a week off or change their routine completely. But if you stop lifting weights entirely, you can expect to lose 50 percent of your newfound strength in two to three months. Your muscle will atrophy (decrease in size), and if you continue to eat as if you are exercising, the excess calories will be stored as fat. So use your muscle or lose it. You really don't want to start over again, do you? Just keep training at an intensity that feels comfortable.

Change your workout every three to four months if you get bored. Replacing one chest exercise for another chest exercise can do this. Another way is to do more repetitions and lessen the load or decrease rest time between sets.

Quality over Quantity

Never sacrifice quality for quantity. Perform each repetition in a smooth and controlled manner, working through the full range of motion that the joint can comfortably go through.

Training speed should be controlled. It is generally recommended that on the difficult aspect (concentric) of the move, take 2–3 seconds; on the easy part (eccentric), take 4–5 seconds. The bottom line is don't do the move super slowly or too fast. Some new research suggests that well-trained older adults may want to perform the moves a little faster to work on the "power aspect" of strength training. Stay alert to this emerging concept.

Do exercises that use the larger muscles of the body (chest and back, front and back of the legs) before moving on to the smaller muscles (arms and calves). When starting out, do compound exercises that employ multiple muscle groups (bench press) over simple, one-muscle exercises (arm curls).

Well-Rounded Program

Remember, strength training should be part of a comprehensive fitness routine that includes cardiovascular fitness (which allows you to walk briskly without getting winded), stretching and flexibility (which allows you to reach down and tie your shoes or zip up your dress without pulling a muscle) and balance work (which prevents you from falling down and breaking a bone). You should also incorporate exercises to improve posture (to allow you to stand with a more upright and youthful carriage) and relaxation (to help you reduce stress and lower your blood pressure).

Greatness lies not in being strong, but in the correct use of strength—therefore, every exercise included in your routine should have a specific purpose or a function. To grow strong, not old and feeble, does not require a great deal of time or expensive equipment or even a membership to a gym. Simply follow the simple steps outlined in this book to achieve this.

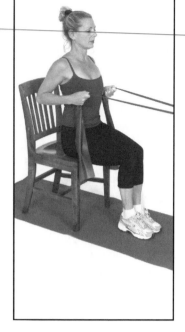

equipment

Strength training can be performed with a variety of equipment: barbells, dumbbells, machines, bands. Which kind you decide to use really has more to do with personal preference and perhaps budget than anything else. Here is a brief list of the pros and cons of each to help you decide on the best equipment for you.

Weights

The type of weights you choose depends on your needs. Luckily, most options are affordable and readily available from the local sporting goods store.

Dumbbells, which come in predetermined weights, are a safe bet. The main drawback is that you usually need several pairs of differing weights in order to effectively work all parts of your body. If you are careful and follow the guidelines in this book, dumbbells are an inexpensive method to improve strength. They can be used in every manner needed to provide a total body workout.

Barbells, a bar that is adjusted by switching out weights on each end of the bar, are a hassle to change and come with a higher risk of injury. Unless you already use barbells regularly, I don't recommend using these.

Ankle weights, which can be strapped on to your ankles or wrists, can make certain exercises easier—and safer—to perform. However, don't strap on the weights as a way to "enhance" leisure activities such as walking, jogging or golfing. Only use them in conjunction with strength exercises.

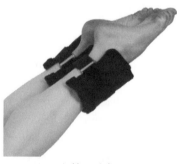
Ankle weights.

Exercise Bands

Every exercise that can be done on a piece of exercise equipment or with weights can be done with an exercise band. They are inexpensive and can

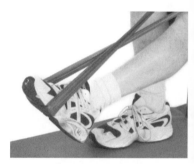
Elastic exercise band.

be stored anywhere. Some even come with handles to hold on to easily.

The bands come in varying resistances. As you get stronger, you may have to purchase more resistant ones in order to accommodate your strength.

Exercise Machines

Exercise machines are an excellent way to improve your strength, but often cannot provide a comprehensive workout. If you have the money to purchase a good-quality multi-station machine, or the time and commitment to attend the gym regularly, that's great. If not, this option is not for you.

My Recommendation

I personally use a combination of dumbbell weights and ankle weights for certain muscle groups and then use exercise bands to complement the rest of the workout. I am also a fan of exercise equipment if you have the space to store it or if you have the money to join a gym. I even use water paddles in the pool to vary my workout on occasion. As discussed earlier, your muscles don't care what is providing the load. You just need to challenge them and change your workout periodically to avoid injury and boredom.

Safety First

No matter which type of equipment you use, always inspect it before using it. Make sure the collars of barbells and dumbbells are on properly, the exercise bands are not worn, and double-check that the cables on machines are in good repair. If you are using a machine, also double-check the weight stack: 100 pounds on one machine is not always 100 pounds on another.

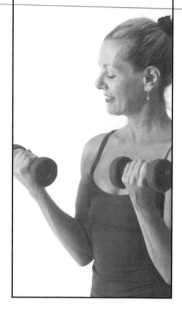

tune into your body

Strength training involves more than hefting a barbell and curling it to your body a few times. In order to keep your body safe and ensure that you're gaining benefits, not injuries, there are several things you must incorporate into your training program. The following are important principles that help you train smart.

Safety

While strength training has numerous benefits, it is not without risk. Even the best exercise can cause pain and injury if done improperly. In the last two decades, it has been reported that nearly a million people have gone to the emergency room for strength-training injuries. A number of injuries are minor but several deaths have occurred from a barbell choking a person who could not lift the bar off their chest or throat. Most of the injuries are the result of over-doing it and not adhering to safe techniques or using outdated principles and exercises. Paying attention to your body can lower your risks of injuring yourself.

While most strength-training exercises will not kill you or even hurt you if done incorrectly once or twice, the cumulative effects can be damaging. Some exercises have been around so long it seems irreverent to question their efficacy. All too often training methods get adopted and later institutionalized based on anecdotal information rather than sound scientific research—what is scientifically acceptable today may not be acceptable tomorrow after further investigation.

Most people understand that physical activity is good for the human machine. Unfortunately, in their zest to get fit they do more than their body is ready to handle. Remember that it is better to train safer and smarter

rather than faster and harder. Think of your 50-plus body as a vintage automobile. A classic car can run just as well as a newer model if well maintained—it just needs a little longer to warm up and more TLC along the way.

Lastly, avoid those well-intended fitness enthusiasts who have all the answers. These people generally base their training methods on popular body-building magazine information rather than scientific information. Stay away from them—these are the people who are going to get you hurt.

Pain

As you get more familiar with strength training, you may

become complacent, and that is when injuries and accidents occur. Learn to listen to your body and trust your ability to distinguish between pain and discomfort.

The old adage "no pain, no gain" is insane. Equally as insane is the adage to work through the pain. Pain is your body telling you that you are doing something wrong. While our bodies are very resilient, misuse, disuse and abuse can cumulate in an injury. Following proper body mechanics and listening to your body can prevent a problem. Prevention is always cheaper than treatment. Protect your spine and joints at all times, and stay mindful of your form.

Posture/Alignment

Think of strength training as adding cement to the forms of a building's foundation. If these forms are not aligned correctly, the building will either be forever crooked or fall apart. The same is true when strength training—always maintain proper alignment. Perfect posture is the key to a symmetrical physique; it also helps you achieve maximum benefits while reducing your risk for injury. Always be mindful of body alignment and proper posture. Avoiding twisting and improper bending. Pay special attention to protect your lower back, knees and shoulders.

Proper Posture

Proper posture is essential in preventing injury and muscular imbalances. Basically, stand with your weight over the balls of your feet and heels, tuck your tailbone between your legs (imagine that you are resting on the edge of a bar stool), make the distance from your

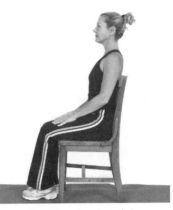

Correct posture in a chair

belly button and your chest as far apart as possible, and pull your belly button in and then place a imaginary apple under your chin. From a side view, your ears, shoulders and hips should be aligned (see the image below). A mental picture that works for my students is to think of your body as a tube of toothpaste, with all the forces squeezing you in and upright.

When sitting, keep your ears aligned over your shoulders and your shoulders aligned over your hips; the knees are aligned over the ankles.

Lower Back

Most of us will experience back pain at some time in our lives. It is critical to protect your back when you strength train. Keep your lower back stable at all times. All back exercises should be done in a slow and controlled manner, and if they increase in discomfort—STOP. Never do exercises in which you bend forward and rotate at

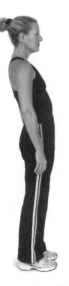
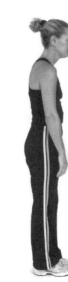
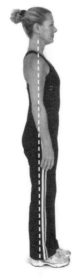
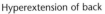

Hyperextension of back   Slouching   Proper posture!

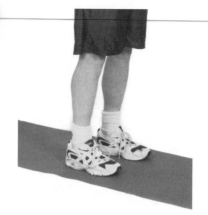

Regular stance

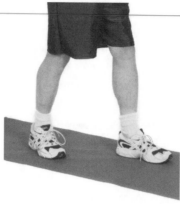

Staggered stance

the same time. Also avoid bending backward at the waist. Quick, uncontrolled trunk twists are not a good idea, either, because torque generated by the twisting action strains the lower back. Be careful when doing fast or forced side bends, too. When sitting on the floor with your legs extended in front of you, be sure to keep your back flat when reaching forward.

Anytime you feel discomfort in your lower back, feel free to adjust your stance (see above). For example, instead of standing with your feet hip-width apart, stand with one foot in front of the other in a comfortable stance.

Shoulders

Shoulder problems are an increasing concern for the over-50 fitness person. Be careful when you bring your arms above your head, and always control any movement that causes you to raise your arms

above shoulder height. Relax your shoulders and don't shrug when you're doing arm exercises. Try your best to keep your shoulder blades pulled together when doing arm moves as well. If your shoulders are tight, don't arch your back to make up for your inflexibility.

Knees

The knees are designed to straighten and bend; any other movement puts them at some level of risk. The knees and toes should always point in

the same direction. Avoid any movements that make your knees rotate or twist, and never twist your body while your feet are planted on the floor. Never straighten your knee so far that it hyperextends, or overly straightens, the leg. Also avoid bending your knees too much. Doing so overstretches the ligaments of the knee and can make the knee joint unstable. Avoid deep knee bends, and make sure you don't squat any lower than the point at which your thighs are parallel to the floor. When lunging, do not allow your knee to extend past your toes. Always remember: Keep your knees "soft" (that is, slightly bent) when strength training. Lastly, don't allow the knee to extend past the toes.

Elbow

When exercising, avoid "locking" or hyperextending your elbow joint. You may cause elbow pain and injury if you do. Keep in mind that the

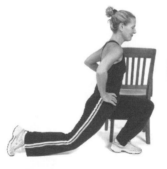

Incorrect: thigh is not parallel to floor and knee is extending beyond the toes

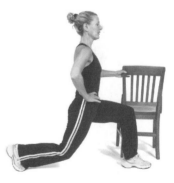

Correct: thigh is parallel to floor and knee is aligned with the ankle

elbow is a "pivot," so in most moves the wrist, elbow and shoulder should be aligned.

Muscular Balance

When performing your workout, think symmetrically. If you do a lot of exercises for your chest, you will notice that your shoulders get rounded. If you work your hamstrings a lot, your quadriceps become weaker in proportion and you will lose flexibility in your legs. Imbalance is the quickest way to injury, so provide balance by exercising both your agonist and antagonist muscle groups. Do unto the front as you do unto the back, and do unto the left as you do unto the right. And remember to stretch what is tight and strengthen what is weak. Keep in mind that you are not just lifting weights to get strong, you are engaging in a body-sculpting activity. When you look at a sculpture of the human body, everything is balanced—no one muscle group is out of proportion. Treat your body like a piece of art.

Breathing

Never hold your breath—doing so while you perform strength-training moves can elevate your blood pressure to dangerous levels. Contrary to popular belief, there is no right or wrong way to breathe. While some trainers suggest that you exhale on effort and inhale on the easy phase, it does not always make sense with certain moves and it does not always feel right with every exercise. The critical aspect is to not hold your breath, whether lifting weights or performing any strenuous maneuver.

Breathe in a manner that feels correct for you, but always include one inhalation and exhalation per repetition. You may want to count out loud or talk while exercising. The key is to breathe freely and effortlessly while strength training.

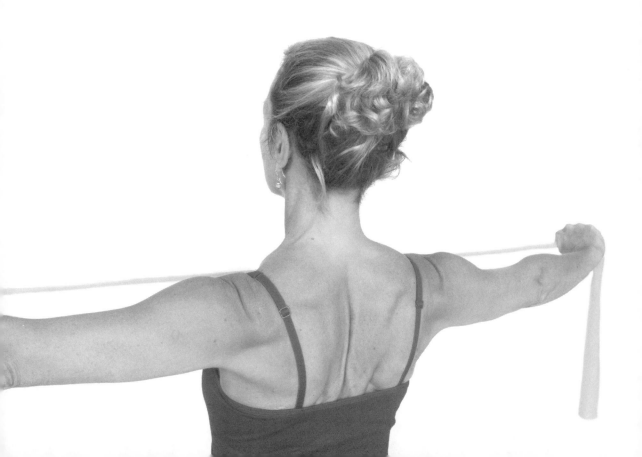

part two:

specialized

programs

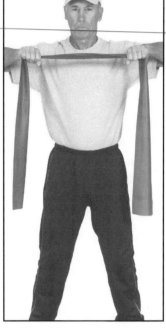

programs overview

By the time many of us turn 50, we may be suffering from twinges in our hinges. The joints affected most frequently are the knees, hips and shoulders, as well as the joints of the lower back. Often these joint issues are the result of abusing or misusing our bodies in our younger days and, unfortunately, may affect our ability to perform daily movements as well as pursue leisure activities. In addition, as we age, our chances of having some type of chronic condition increases.

In the U.S., millions of people over 50 years of age have a chronic condition such as diabetes, cancer, heart disease, stroke, hypertension and/or arthritis. This section provides strength-training programs to help improve many chronic conditions seen in the 50-plus group, as well as make recreational pursuits easier.

Warm Up First, Stretch After

It is best to warm up the muscles you plan to use with active stretches and a light jog or five-minute-long walk prior to doing any activity. Treat yourself like an expensive racehorse—no horse owner would ever allow the horse to go out on the track without being completely warmed up. So don't do anything, from shoveling snow to golfing, without warming up your body first. Note that warming up is not the same as stretching! Slowly and mindfully do a few minutes of light activity before strength training, attending to your daily chores or doing your favorite sport.

Once you're done with your strength training, remember to stretch the muscles you've used. This will help your body release any accumulated tension or tightness.

Fit Tips

• Always obtain medical clearance before starting. Ask your doctor about recommendations regarding exercise heart rates and exercise blood pressure levels, as well as other suggestions and cautions. If your blood pressure is over 160/90 before you exercise, don't exercise that day until you consult your physician.

EXERCISE CAUTIONS

Stop exercising and call 911 immediately if you experience any of the following:

- Chest pain, arm pain or tightness in the chest, neck, throat
- Difficulty breathing
- Abnormal heart rhythm
- Light-headedness
- Visual changes
- Numbness in the face or limbs
- Extreme weakness
- Excessive cold sweat
- If you cannot repeat a simple sentence and smile while holding your arms up in the air (you may be experiencing a stroke)

- Dress in layers in order to peel off clothes after you warm up.
- Always warm up before and cool down/stretch after each exercise session. I've suggested appropriate stretches for each workout.
- Feel free to do some or all of the suggested exercises. Just remember to listen to your body—if your shoulder is bothering you one day, skip the shoulder exercises but train another part of the body instead.
- Exercise at a pace and intensity that makes you feel good.
- Stop anytime you feel pain—do not try to work through the pain!
- Keep in mind the two-hour rule: If you hurt significantly more two hours post-exercise, ease off to an intensity that does not provoke any discomfort. But don't quit.
- Expect setbacks—don't get discouraged. There will be times when you don't want to exercise, which is normal, but rather than not exercising that day, just do a little. It is okay to just do your favorite exercises. If after 5-10 minutes you still don't feel good, skip your exercise for that day. However, if you are running a fever, injured or sick, take a day off.
- The hardest part of any exercise program is just doing it. Negative self-talk will destroy your intentions to improve your health. Set yourself up to be successful. Don't let people sabotage your efforts. Be a fitness achiever, not a fitness drop-out.

Aerobic Suggestions

Although this book focuses on strength training, aerobic exercise is essential in keeping your body in good working order.

Many individuals with arthritis and other chronic conditions complement their strength training with an aerobic workout in the water, whether it be swimming or water exercise. Riding a stationary bike is another option; recumbent bikes provide back support for those who need it.

Walking can be done anywhere, anytime. Be sure you have good shoes and, at first, take in short distances to see how your body and joints feel. Walking on a soft track is often easier on the back, knees and ankles than the hard sidewalk. Many treadmills provide excellent cushion while walking. Avoid jogging.

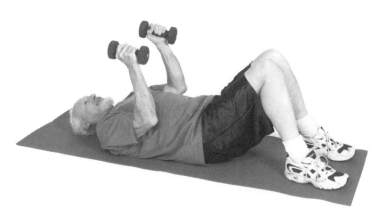

chronic conditions

A chronic condition, unlike an acute health issue, usually cannot be cured. Often, it has an uncertain outcome and at best can only be managed for the remainder of the person's life. Another aspect of a chronic condition is that it permeates the person's lifestyle both financially and medically, as well as affects interpersonal relationships.

Physical therapists, exercise physiologists and other experts in the field of older adult fitness agree that most of the chronic conditions seen in the over-50 population, from arthritis to Parkinson's disease, can be positively influenced with regular and sensible strength training. Strength training has been found to reduce lower back pain, improve leg function in people with bad knees, and help those with heart problems be better able to meet the demands of daily living.

Regardless of our age or physical condition, improvements in muscular strength can play a pivotal role in reducing the amount of disability we have. The focus on strength training for individuals with chronic conditions should be on fostering functional and independent living skills—*not*

exacerbating their existing condition. That's what the programs in this section strive to do.

Don't Be Limited by Your Limitations

In order to overcome a chronic condition, think about the benefits of your successes rather than the consequences of your failures. Too many people give up on an exercise program long before they experience the benefits that regular exercise can provide. Increased strength often translates into better functional fitness that will improve your ability to participate more fully in the mainstream of life and reduce the burden on your caregiver, if you have one. More importantly, strength training empowers the person with a chronic condition to live a richer and fuller life.

Decide what you want as an end product of your exercise program and then design it to match your goals and abilities. Be your own personal trainer. Make your life and your body the best they can be. When exercise is done properly and prudently, good outcomes are generally derived. Regular exercise is therapy for the mind and body. Remember that you are the captain of your wellness

ship and no one truly cares more about you than you! Your doctor and your family can be cheerleaders but you are the captain.

General Guidelines

- Always consult your health professional about suggestions regarding exercise and your condition. Information in this section is not a substitute for medical advice.
- Perform your exercise program when you are having the least amount of pain/discomfort. Avoid exercising on days when you are experiencing a flare up.
- If you are exercising alone, carry ID and medical information with you.
- Be mindful of doing the movement with the best pain-free technique you can do. If it hurts—STOP! Also stop if the amount of pain you experience increases both during and after. Exercise should be pain-free.
- Never hold your breath.
- If you exercise alone, keep a phone handy.

Arthritis

There are more than 100 forms of arthritis. Stiffness and chronic pain are common characteristics. The phrase "use it or lose it" really applies to arthritis: if you don't move that joint, it will become stiffer and weaker. Unfortunately, many people with arthritis are afraid to exercise in fear that they will make the condition worst. Thus the downward spiral begins: As the person with arthritis starts to do less, the muscles weaken, which in turn puts more load and strain on an already compromised joint.

A mild to moderate strength-training routine can go a long way in preventing further atrophy of the muscle that supports the joint. It also increases muscle tone and strength, which adds integrity to the joint, and helps maintain or increases bone strength. The goal of this strength program is to maximize benefits and minimize risks, so always consult with your doctor or therapist before starting a routine. Learn what kind of arthritis you have and what kind of exercise is best for your condition.

No matter what type of arthritis you have, it is critical that you do not cause any further harm to the joint—train the muscles, don't strain the joints. Also, do everything you can to prevent additional pain, but do not increase your medications to cover up pain. I've suggested some stretches to increase range of motion.

Guidelines

- Avoid extremes in motion of flexion and extension.
- Avoid jarring and twisting motions.

chronic conditions

ARTHRITIS

	PAGE	EXERCISE
	116	elbow touches
	125	rear calf stretch
	121	seated knee to chest
	61	quad setting
	56	seated leg extensions
	65	leg curls
	102	biceps curls
	93	shrugs

Back Pain

Lower back pain is caused by a variety of sources: weak abdominal muscles, improper body mechanics, poor posture, overuse, facet and joint problems along with herniated discs. Since there are many causes, always consult a health professional for a proper diagnosis.

It is also a good idea to have a physical therapist show you how to stand properly and teach you proper body mechanics for daily life activities so as not to exacerbate your condition any further. Core training stabilizes and supports the spine by strengthening the muscles that surround the spine and torso, commonly called the "core." It's much like building your own internal back brace. Think of your body as a sunflower: develop a solid stem to hold the flower tall. See page 23 for a brief lesson on how to stand and sit properly.

Most back issues can be improved with a sound exercise program using proper body mechanics. However, avoid overdoing it and performing questionable moves. Once a person has had a back problem, it is likely to occur again.

Guidelines
• If you notice an increase in pain and/or numbness in your legs or feet, stop and see your health professional.

• Avoid movements that increase the load on your spine, such as the Military Press and bending over at the waist.

chronic conditions

BACK PAIN

	PAGE	EXERCISE
	73	bicycle
	71	curl-ups
	76	buttocks lifts
	77	pointer
	83	incline presses
	96	military presses with band
	90	shoulder retractions
	113	triceps band extensions
	123	sit & reach
	121	seated knee to chest
	124	figure 4

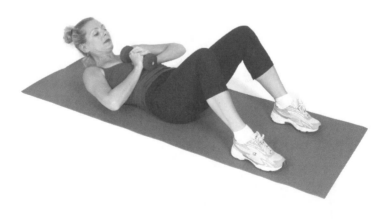

Breathing Conditions

Chronic obstructive pulmonary disease (COPD) is a progressive disorder of the lungs characterized by the destruction of the alveoli, retention of mucus secretions and so on. Common conditions grouped under this heading include bronchitis, asthma, emphysema and sometime allergies—all of which make breathing difficult. It is common to see individuals who have COPD not engage in much activity. Research shows that a slow, progressive overall fitness program often leads to better aerobic fitness, which in turn leads to a better quality of life.

A gentle strength-training program with several rest breaks is the first step toward reversing the downward spiral often associated with COPD. The goal of strength training is to improve the muscles of the legs that make getting up and down from a chair easier, as well as being able to move around without getting short of breath. This program will also

chronic conditions

	PAGE	EXERCISE
	90	shoulder retractions
	91	bow & arrow
	93	shrugs
	55	sit to stand
	56	seated leg extensions
	116	elbow touches

BREATHING CONDITIONS

improve ventilation, improve strength and endurance of respiratory muscles, maintain and improve chest and back mobility, improve leg strength to make activities of daily living easier, and teach effective breathing patterns.

Guidelines

• Start very, very slow. Avoid getting out of breath.
• Never overextend yourself. It is better to do 1–2 minutes of exercise, rest and then repeat your bout of exercise than it is to try to work up to 10-15 minutes of non-stop exercise.
• Learn how to do "pursed-lip breathing" from your health care provider and follow their recommendations. If you use an inhaler, consult your doctor about exercising and the use of the device.

Diabetes

There are two types of diabetes mellitus: juvenile diabetes, or type 1 diabetes, and adult-onset diabetes, or type 2 diabetes. When a person has diabetes, the body does not provide enough of the hormone insulin, which helps regulate the amount of sugar in the blood stream.

Regular exercise can help a person with diabetes stabilize the condition. Having diabetes or being at risk for developing diabetes is not an excuse not to exercise but rather a reason to exercise. As with any other chronic condition, prior to starting an exercise program consult your health professional for any special recommendations and precautions specific to you.

Flexibility training is another important aspect of training for someone with diabetes. For additional stretches, see *Stretching for 50+*.

Guidelines

- Set a goal of performing at least 30 minutes of aerobic exercise most days of the week at a comfortable pace. If you are unable to do 30 minutes of non-stop exercise, it is okay to break it up into three bouts of 10 minutes each.
- Avoid activities that are stressful to your feet.
- Extended warm-up and cool-

chronic conditions

DIABETES

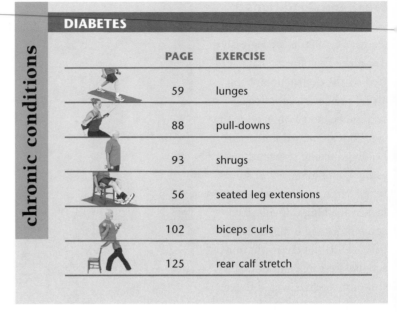

	PAGE	EXERCISE
	59	lunges
	88	pull-downs
	93	shrugs
	56	seated leg extensions
	102	biceps curls
	125	rear calf stretch

down periods are important for diabetics when transitioning from moderate exercise to rest.
- Perform strength-training loads that are not strenuous. Do 10–15 reps with a light to moderate load. If you have diabetic retinopathy, avoid intense exercise such as lifting heavy weights.
- Train at a heart rate that is less than someone who does not have diabetes. Train, don't strain.
- Consult your health professional about which insulin level and glucose level is right for you. Keep some hard candy or easily digestible carbohydrate available should you need it.
- Exercise at predictable times to minimize blood sugar fluctuations.

- Be alert to signs of hypoglycemia and diabetic coma.
- Drink fluids regularly.
- Monitor your blood pressure levels (consult your doctor regarding this matter).
- If you are injecting insulin, be mindful of where the injection is and what set of muscles you are planning to use. Discuss with your health professional about appropriate injection sites when exercising. A general tip is not to inject the area that you will be exercising that day.

Don't exercise if you have:
- Retinal hemorrhages
- Fever or infection
- Very low or very high blood glucose levels (consult your doctor for specific details).

Heart Issues

Heart disease, the leading cause of death for both men and women in the United States, includes such things as high blood pressure, arteriosclerosis, coronary artery disease, angina, and congestive heart disease. Fit people have less heart disease than do less fit individuals. A sensible and medically approved exercise program, along with modifications in diet and stress levels, will improve the quality of life. If you have had a heart attack or stroke, it is prudent to attend a medically supervised exercise program before exercising on your own.

Many people who have suffered a heart attack are afraid to live for fear of dying. This can often be more devastating than the heart attack itself, which is why a regular fitness routine is so critical to the person who wants to fully engage in the mainstream of life once more. Strength training should only be added after a baseline

chronic conditions

HEART ISSUES		
	PAGE	EXERCISE
	80	chair push-ups
	55	sit to stand
	60	leg presses
	65	leg curls
	102	biceps curls
	113	triceps band extensions

of fitness has been achieved and your doctor has given you permission to do so. Strength training can help activities of daily living become less strenuous. In addition to engaging in a sensible exercise program, a healthy lifestyle must be adopted: stop smoking; eat right and eat lean; reduce stress; exercise aerobically; follow your doctor's recommendations and take your medications as directed.

Guidelines

- If you are on a beta-blocker or similar medication to "cap" your heart rate, use the "talk test" to determine your intensity: If you can't talk easily, then you are working too hard—slow down.
- Slow and steady wins the race: avoid exercising hard and fast. You are exercising for your life—don't put it at risk while exercising.

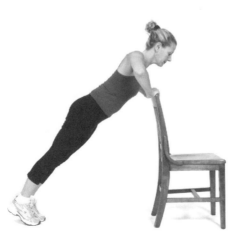

High Blood Pressure

It is believed that high blood pressure (hypertension) is the third most common chronic condition in the United States, right behind sinusitis and arthritis. Your blood pressure fluctuates from moment to moment and is affected by everything from stress and environmental stimulation to physical exertion. High blood pressure is a major risk factor in developing a stroke, heart disease and several other health issues. High blood pressure is often called the silent killer since it does not manifest any outward symptoms until either you die, have a stroke or have a heart attack. Always monitor your blood pressure! It is wise to ask your doctor if resistance training is okay for you before starting.

The first approach to improving blood pressure is lifestyle changes that include diet, stress management and regular exercise. Numerous studies have shown that aerobic exercise has a positive influence on lowering blood

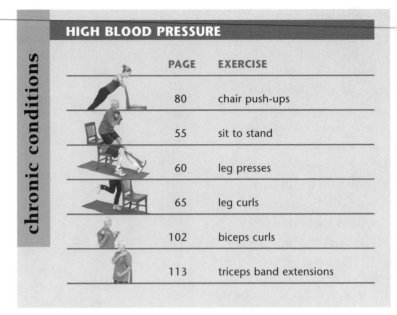

chronic conditions

HIGH BLOOD PRESSURE

	PAGE	EXERCISE
	80	chair push-ups
	55	sit to stand
	60	leg presses
	65	leg curls
	102	biceps curls
	113	triceps band extensions

pressure. Use caution if you choose to strength training. Strength training can elevate your blood pressure to dangerous levels; therefore, consult your doctor before doing any strength-training moves.

Guidelines

- Avoid heavy strength training. Performing higher reps with lightweights is a better way to go.
- If your blood pressure is above 160/90, check with your doctor before lifting weights.
- Be careful of overhead lifts.
- Always make time to adequately warm up and cool down. People with vascular issues such as high or low blood pressure can get into trouble if they start out too hard and stop exercising abruptly.
- Emphasize muscular endurance over strength and power. The goal should be to do a higher number of reps rather than less reps with a heavier load.

Knee Problems

Chronic knee problems can be the result of poor anatomical design. For example, being knock-kneed and bowlegged can set you up for injury. Simple activities such as jogging or even walking can increase the load on the knee joint three to five times the person's body weight. In addition, sports injuries from soccer, football or even biking with poor form can harm your knees. The causes of knee problems are many and range from arthritis to misuse and abuse. See your doctor to get a proper diagnosis and corrective suggestions. To reduce knee pain, strengthen all the muscles of your quads, and remember that exercise should not increase pain or swelling.

Guidelines

- Always point your toes and knees in the same direction.
- Never go past your safe range of motion.
- Avoid over-straightening your legs.
- If you are told to wear a brace when exercising, be sure to follow all recommendations.
- Ice your knee after exercise, if recommended.
- Wear good supportive shoes and replace them every 500 miles or three to six months.

chronic conditions

KNEE PROBLEMS

	PAGE	EXERCISE
	61	quad setting
	64	wall squats
	60	leg presses
	56	seated leg extensions
	59	lunges
	65	leg curls
	125	rear calf stretch

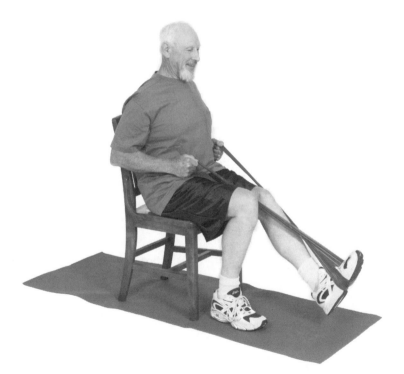

Osteoporosis

Osteoporosis is a significant loss of bone mass that leads to increased porosity, making the bone more at risk for a fracture. One of the leading risk factors is lack of regular weight-bearing exercise. Osteoporosis is a silent disease; the first sign of it is often a fracture. A turn can cause the hip joint to snap; a simple fall can result in a fracture of the wrist or, even worse, a broken hip.

Fortunately, osteoporosis is not inevitable. It is never to late for action. Your bones are living structures that are re-modeling themselves everyday. Along with sound lifestyle choices, resistance-training exercise can minimize the weakening of your bones. Wolfe's law says that "the robustness of the bone is directly related to the forces applied to it." In other words, your bones are what you make of them. If you lead a sedentary life, you will have bones designed for easy living; if, on the other hand, you challenge your bones, you will have bones better prepared for an occasional tumble. Additionally, if you make your muscles stronger, the research shows

that the bones will get stronger too. Also, if you get stronger, maybe you will be strong enough to catch your balance and not fall. If you only have osteopenia now, by beginning strength training right now you may be able to prevent yourself from ever developing full-blown osteoporosis.

Strength-training exercises have been shown to improve balance and gait, improve flexibility and reverse muscle atrophy, which can prevent falls. Strength training also places good stresses on bones that will stimulate thickness of the bones and improve their density.

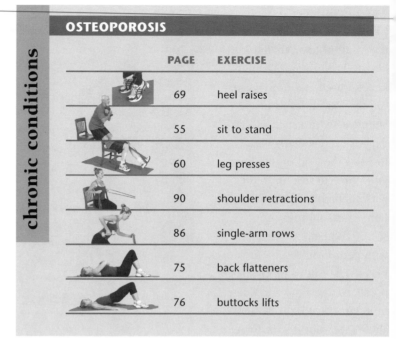

chronic conditions

OSTEOPOROSIS

PAGE	EXERCISE
69	heel raises
55	sit to stand
60	leg presses
90	shoulder retractions
86	single-arm rows
75	back flatteners
76	buttocks lifts

Exercise Contraindications

While exercise has been proven to improve bone density, certain exercises could cause a compression fracture. Therefore, avoid the following moves:

- Bent over rowing
- Overhead lifts with weights
- Twisting moves
- Squats with a load placed on your shoulders or any exercise that places a load down on your spine
- Heavy-impact moves

Shoulder Problems

The design of the shoulder is remarkable, allowing a baseball pitcher to throw a ball 90 mph or allowing a person to rock a baby to sleep. The shoulder is a ball and socket joint that gets its support from muscles, ligaments and tendons. Some experts believe that when you move your arm, as many as 26 muscles are engaged at some time in the movement. The more active you are, the greater the risk of injuring your shoulder. It is common to see adults over 50 years of age suffer from a shoulder condition as they get older. Shoulder problems can be the result of many things, including bursitis and tendonitis; or they can be idiopathic (i.e., no known cause).

Many times the corrective exercises will be the same regardless of the cause. But it is still wise to have a medical doctor provide you with a proper diagnosis and have a physical therapist give you corrective exercises. Some of the common conditions seen in the older adult population are rotator cuff injury and frozen shoulder. Stretching is very important for people with shoulder problems—I've included some in this workout.

Exercise Contraindications

Avoid overhead arm exercises or any moves that increase pain and/or limit your range of motion.

SHOULDER PROBLEMS

	PAGE	EXERCISE
	100	internal rotations
	101	external rotations
	87	reverse band flyes
	93	shrugs
	98	sword fighter
	99	reverse sword fighter
	88	pull-downs
	115	soup can pours
	91	bow & arrow
	118	choker
	117	over the top

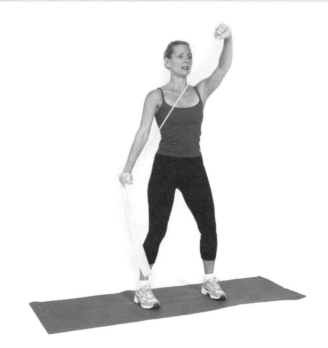

recreational pursuits

Many sports and recreational pursuits require the body to perform the same movement over and over again, causing overuse syndrome and the adaptive shortening of a muscle. Strength training for recreational pursuits has several functions. It reverses the muscle imbalances caused by repetitive movements and it strengthens the muscle so that it can handle the stress placed on it when training. In this sense, strength training prevents possible injuries. A well-conditioned muscle easily outperforms a weak or unconditioned muscle. Here are some workouts for popular activities.

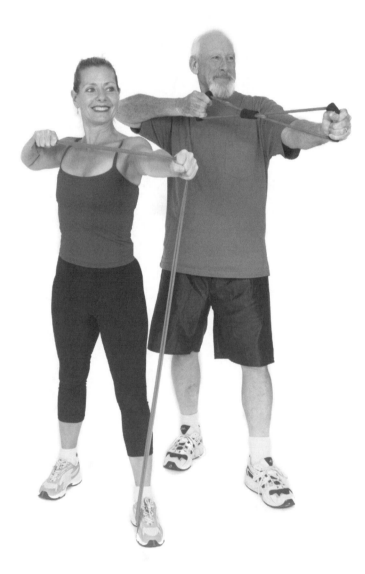

Biking

Most people assume that biking is solely a lower body activity. But think about your posture: your body hunches over the handlebars, with much of your weight resting on your wrists and hands. While biking does primarily engage the lower body, requiring muscular endurance and strength of the legs and stamina of the lower back, a person needs enough strength to support the upper body and head.

A fitness program for cycling conditions all the muscles of the leg in addition to correcting the muscles of the body that are fostering poor posture. The bottom line is to increase the strength and endurance of the lower extremities by performing higher reps, as well as condition the upper body to counteract any muscular imbalances caused by cycling.

recreational pursuits

BIKING

	PAGE	EXERCISE
	59	lunges
	67	hands and knees leg curls
	62	single-leg squats
	57	standing leg extensions
	94	lateral arm raises
	85	prone reverse flyes
	87	reverse band flyes
	90	shoulder retractions
	71	curl-ups
	76	buttocks lifts
	125	rear calf stretch
	119	pec stretch
	122	double knee to chest

ADVANCED ADDITIONS

	PAGE	EXERCISE
	82	band push-ups
	111	chair dips 1
	112	chair dips 2

Bowling

Many people don't think of bowling as a sport, yet it can be very hard on the lower back, hips and shoulders. Bowling is a one-sided activity that requires you to throw a heavy ball with significant force to knock over the pins. This can cause muscle imbalances, which can lead to injury. Strength training can help to correct many of these issues by strengthening the total body as well as improving flexibility. Since bowling is an activity that requires strength and power, you should work towards improving both. Therefore, once you establish a baseline of muscular strength and endurance, start focusing on doing moves more quickly. However, keep in mind that explosive moves put you at more risk for injury, so train smart, not hard.

recreational pursuits

BOWLING

	PAGE	EXERCISE
	104	cross-your-heart curls
	105	concentration curls
	106	reverse curls
	107	wrist curls
	59	lunges
	72	curl-ups with a twist
	63	downhill skier
	118	choker
	121	seated knee to chest
	125	rear calf stretch

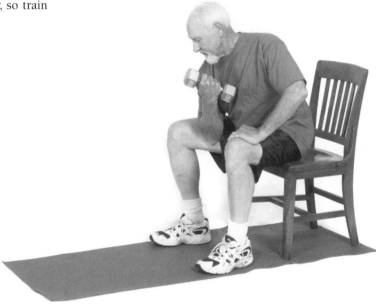

Golf

Many people say they play golf, yet I am still waiting to meet someone who actually "plays" golf. Most people compete at golf, either against others or themselves. Golf is a tough game on the body, requiring twisting of the knees and lower back. This asymmetrical sport, with moves repeated sometimes up to 90 times, presents a whole set of problems. Ironically, the worse you are at the game, the harder it is on your body because you take more swings—with biomechanically incorrect form.

A golfer does not require big muscles or a lot of strength, but the game requires controlled power. Therefore, your exercise program should try to replicate the moves and the speed used on the course. But for your health, a sound fitness program should be aimed at undoing the unilateral movement. Work all the muscles of the body and keep the body fluid. Stretch what is tight and inflexible and strengthen what is weak. After you develop a baseline of strength, increase your power by doing the moves more quickly. However, be careful—ballistic moves can cause injuries.

recreational pursuits

GOLF

	PAGE	EXERCISE
	107	wrist curls
	106	reverse curls
	101	external rotations
	100	internal rotations
	80	chair push-ups
	88	pull-downs
	75	back flatteners
	78	dumbbell presses
	79	dumbbell flyes
	51	leg squeeze & spread
	125	rear calf stretch
	123	sit & reach
	121	seated knee to chest
	115	soup can pours

Jogging/Walking

Walking and jogging are excellent aerobic activities that, unfortunately, stress the lower limbs by placing three to five times your body weight on your knees. However, the muscles of the torso are engaged as well, so when designing your routine, place most of your focus on upper body conditioning and stretching the muscles of the lower body and back. Focus on muscular endurance more than strength and power. A strength program for a walker/jogger will be aimed at higher reps with lighter load.

recreational pursuits

JOGGING/WALKING

	PAGE	EXERCISE
	93	shrugs
	98	sword fighter
	92	seated rows
	83	incline presses
	103	hammer curls
	108	side-lying triceps extensions
	71	curl-ups
	76	buttocks lifts
	58	straight-leg lifts
	64	wall squats
	69	heel raises
	125	rear calf stretch
	123	sit & reach
	116	elbow touches

stretches

ADVANCED ADDITIONS

	PAGE	EXERCISE
	82	band push-ups
	111	chair dips 1
	112	chair dips 2

Swimming

Although swimming does not provide much challenge for the bones of the body, it is an excellent way to improve cardiovascular fitness. However, people mistakenly believe that swimming is a gentle way to get fit. In fact, swimming can be hard on the shoulders and even the neck and lower back if your form is faulty. Another problem arises if you don't vary your strokes—all the muscles on the front of your body get worked (and consequently get tight) while your upper back becomes hunched over

If you are a competitive swimmer, you need to focus on improving your muscular endurance. If you are swimming for health and fitness, you'll want to improve muscular strength, challenge the bones of the body by doing weight-bearing exercises and reverse hunched-over posture. When designing your routine, the bottom line is to stretch what is tight and inflexible and strengthen what is weak.

recreational pursuits

SWIMMING

	PAGE	EXERCISE
	109	bent-over triceps extensions
	95	frontal arm raises
	97	upright rows
	99	reverse sword fighter
	88	pull-downs
	83	incline presses
	87	reverse band flyes
	55	sit to stand
	65	leg curls
	59	lunges
	115	soup can pours
	116	elbow touches
	119	pec stretch
	120	zipper

Skiing

Skiing, whether cross-country or downhill, requires good lower body strength and endurance. You also have to contend with cold weather and high altitudes—generally, the muscles, tendons and ligaments over people over 50 often gel up under these circumstances. Skiing is a total body sport that can be hard on the shoulders and the knees.

Downhill skiing is explosive, asking you to work hard for short periods of time, while cross-country skiing requires good muscular endurance. Both forms of skiing also place high demands on the upper body when using your poles either to plant for a turn or pull. This sport, maybe more than any other, insists that you be in fine shape if you plan to ski aggressively. This sport demands that you be well conditioned before you make your trek up the mountain, thus your training routine should start long before you plan to ski. This sport is a sport where specificity of training is required. The routine for cross-country skiing are much different than downhill skiing. However, both require a baseline of cardiovascular fitness and an ok by the doctor before embarking to the mountains.

The purpose of this strength-training program is to give you a total body workout that addresses muscular power and endurance.

recreational pursuits

DOWNHILL SKIING

	PAGE	EXERCISE
	114	horizontal triceps extensions
	95	frontal arm raises
	96	military presses with band
	84	high flyes
	89	y pull-downs
	52	side lunges
	63	downhill skier
	53	side-lying leg raises
	64	wall squats
	65	leg curls

CROSS-COUNTRY SKIING

	PAGE	EXERCISE
	102	biceps curls
	110	supine triceps extensions
	95	frontal arm raises
	92	seated rows
	52	side lunges
	53	side-lying leg raises
	54	reverse side-lying leg raises
	59	lunges
	65	leg curls

Tennis

Tennis is fun but can take its toll on the lower body, shoulders and elbows. The knees take a pounding and also make quick turns and twists. The shoulders reach and stretch in all directions and respond with speed and power. The load placed upon the back, not to mention the cardiovascular system, is tremendous. Additionally, for most people tennis is a one-sided sport, further contributing to physical problems. Many people over 50 find that a singles game of tennis is more than they want to engage in and opt for a friendly game of doubles.

The following strength program gives you enough strength to continue playing. Since tennis is an explosive sport that requires bursts of speed and power, once you establish a baseline of muscular strength and endurance, your program should start focusing on developing power by doing moves more quickly. However, keep in mind that explosive moves put you at more risk for injury, so train smart, not hard. But most important and critical for the health of your body is a total comprehensive fitness program that includes exercising all the muscles of the body, regular stretching and aerobic work.

recreational pursuits

TENNIS

PAGE	EXERCISE
104	cross-your-heart curls
106	reverse curls
114	horizontal triceps extensions
98	sword fighter
100	internal rotations
101	external rotations
81	baby boomer push-ups
73	bicycle
76	buttocks lifts
74	marching
52	side lunges
66	prone leg curls
59	lunges
68	gas pedals
50	standing leg raises
70	one-leg heel raises
125	rear calf stretch
115	soup can pours
119	pec stretch
123	sit & reach
122	double knee to chest

part three:

the exercises

standing leg raises

starting position

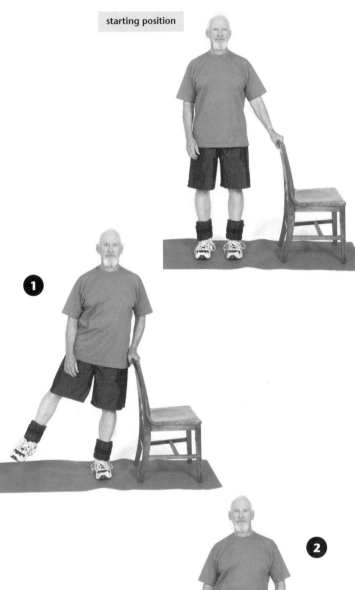

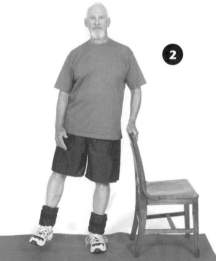

If you find this exercise too difficult, try it without weights.

STARTING POSITION: Strap an ankle weight around each ankle and stand with proper posture. Place your left hand on a stable chair for balance. **INHALE** to begin.

1 Keeping your foot pointed forward, **EXHALE** and slowly raise the outside leg out to the side as high as is comfortable and hold.

2 **INHALE** and slowly return to starting position with control.

Repeat, then switch sides.

VARIATION

To perform this with an exercise band, tie the ends of the band together and loop it around both ankles.

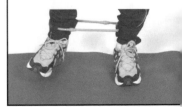

leg squeeze & spread

target: inner & outer thighs

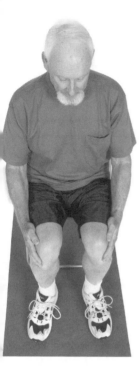

starting position

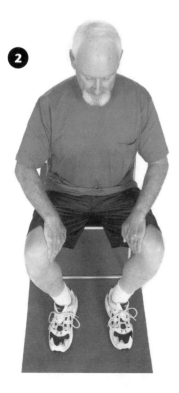

Do not apply too much resistance with either of these steps.

STARTING POSITION: Sit toward the front of a chair with both feet flat on the floor. Place your hands on the outsides of your thighs near your knees. Breathe comfortably.

1 Spread your legs a comfortable width as you resist the motion with your hands.

2 Now place your hands on the insides of your thighs and resist the motion as you squeeze your legs together.

side lunges

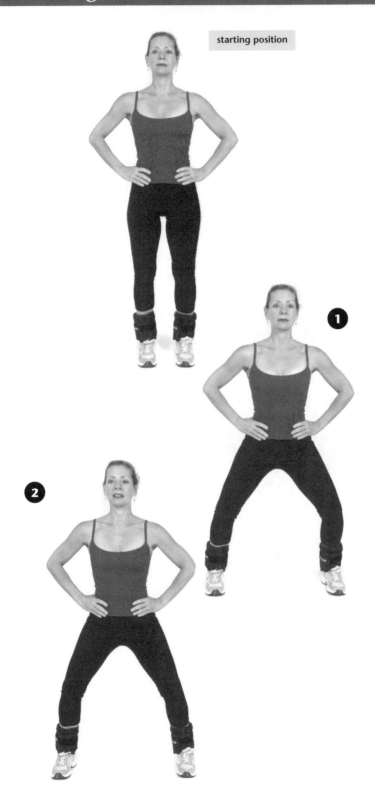

starting position

This is a very advanced move and requires excellent balance. Beginners can hold onto a chair for balance or try this without weights.

STARTING POSITION: Strap an ankle weight around each ankle and stand with proper posture, hands on your hips. **INHALE** to begin.

1 **EXHALE** and slowly step out to the left side, making sure your knees don't go past your toes. **INHALE** to return to starting position.

3 **EXHALE** and slowly step out to the right side. **INHALE** to return to starting position.

VARIATION

As this moves becomes easy, you can step out to the side and perform a quarter squat.

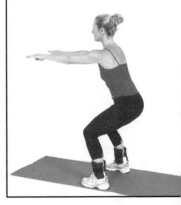

side-lying leg raises

target: outer thighs

starting position

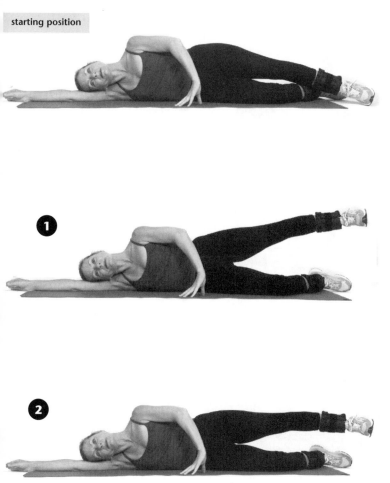

If you find this exercise too difficult, try it without weights.

STARTING POSITION: Strap an ankle weight around each ankle and lie on the right side of your body, positioning your body in a comfortable position so as to not hurt your back. You can bend your lower leg to reduce stress on your back. Rest your head on your right upper arm and straighten the top leg. **INHALE** to begin.

1 Keeping your left leg straight, **EXHALE** and lift it up to shoulder height.

2 **INHALE** and slowly return to starting position.

Repeat, then switch sides.

VARIATION

To perform this with an exercise band, tie the ends of the band together and loop it around both ankles.

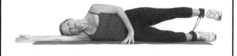

reverse side-lying leg raises

starting position

If you find this exercise too difficult, try it without weights.

STARTING POSITION: Strap an ankle weight around each ankle and lie on the right side of your body. Rest your head on your right upper arm and straighten the lower leg. Bend your top leg and place the foot over and in front of your other leg; try to keep this foot flat on the floor. Place your other hand on the floor in front of your pelvis for support. **INHALE** to begin.

1 Keeping your lower leg straight, **EXHALE** and lift it as high as is comfortable and hold.

2 **INHALE** and lower to starting position.

Repeat, then switch sides.

sit to stand

target: quadriceps

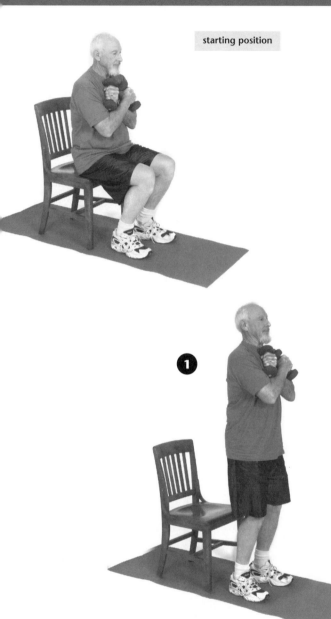

starting position

If you find this exercise too difficult, try it without weights.

STARTING POSITION: Sit toward the front of a sturdy chair, placing your feet flat on the floor, just slightly behind your knees. Hold a dumbbell in each hand and cross your arms in front of your chest. Lean slightly forward and keep your torso firm as you perform this exercise. **INHALE** to begin.

1 **EXHALE** and slowly stand up without using your hands, if possible.

2 **INHALE** and lower yourself slowly into the chair.

starting position

If you have long legs, roll up a towel and place it under your knees to raise them. If you find this exercise too difficult, try it without weights.

STARTING POSITION: Strap an ankle weight to each ankle and sit with your back against the back of the chair. Place your hands in a comfortable position. **INHALE** to begin.

1 **EXHALE** and slowly extend your right leg until it's straight, but not hyperextended. Hold for a count of 1-2.

2 **INHALE** and slowly return your leg to starting position.

Repeat, then switch sides.

1

2

starting position

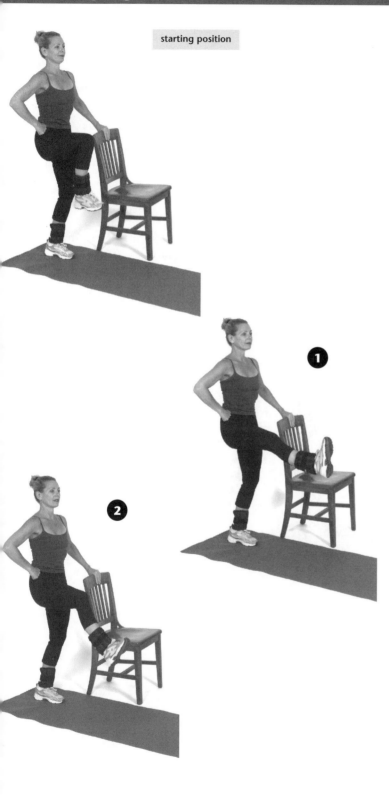

1

2

If you find this exercise too difficult, try it without weights.

STARTING POSITION: Strap an ankle weight to each ankle and stand with proper posture next to a sturdy chair. Lift your right thigh in front of you as high as is comfortable (but no higher than parallel with the floor). **INHALE** to begin.

1 **EXHALE** and slowly extend (kick) your right foot forward until it is fully extended. Hold for a count of 1-2.

2 **INHALE** and slowly return your leg to starting position.

Repeat, then switch sides.

MODIFICATION

If you are not strong enough to hold the leg up unsupported, it is okay to use your hands to help keep the leg up.

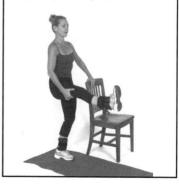

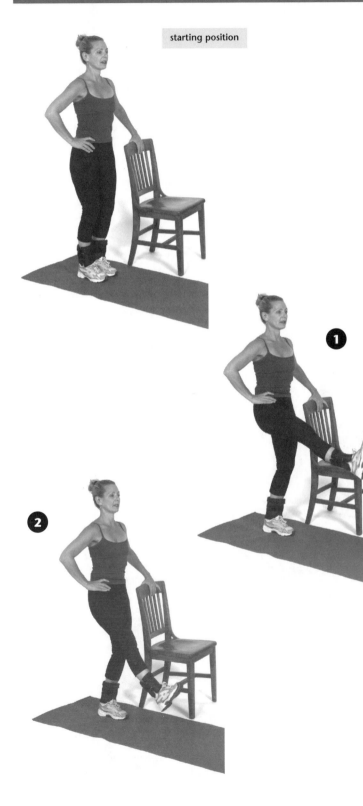

starting position

If you find this exercise too difficult, try it without weights.

STARTING POSITION: Strap an ankle weight to each ankle and stand next to a sturdy chair. Maintain proper posture throughout the movement. **INHALE** to begin.

1 **EXHALE** and straighten your outside leg and move it forward as high as is comfortable. Make sure you don't lean back while you raise your leg.

2 **INHALE** and slowly return to starting position.

Repeat, then switch sides.

lunges

target: quadriceps

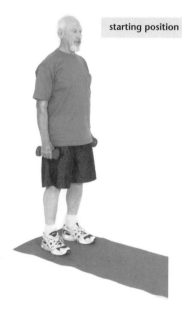

starting position

If you find this too difficult, do this movement without weights and place your hands on your hips instead.

STARTING POSITION: Stand with proper posture and hold a dumbbell in each hand by your sides. **INHALE** to begin.

1 Keeping your left leg in place, **EXHALE** and lunge forward with your right leg as far as is comfortable, but keeping your knee in line with your ankle.

2 **INHALE** as you step back to starting position.

Repeat, then switch sides.

1

2

MODIFICATION

If balance is an issue, hold a dumbbell in one hand and hold onto a chair with your free hand.

VARIATION

As your balance and strength improve, alternate legs with each lunge rather than doing all reps on one side.

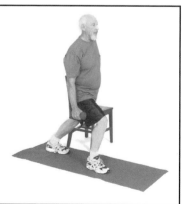

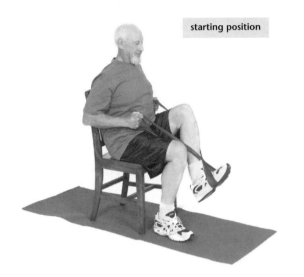

starting position

STARTING POSITION: Sit with proper posture in the middle of the chair. Wrap the exercise band around your left foot once and hold on to the ends of the band. **INHALE** to begin.

1 **EXHALE** and slowly extend your left leg forward, but do not lock your knee.

2 **INHALE** and slowly return to starting position.

Repeat, then switch sides.

❶

❷

starting position

If you find this exercise too difficult, try it without weights.

STARTING POSITION: Strap an ankle weight to each ankle and sit in a chair with proper posture. Straighten your right leg by tightening the upper leg muscles. **INHALE** to begin.

1 Keep your right leg straight as you **EXHALE** and lift it up so that it's parallel with the floor. Do not lean back as you lift your leg.

2 **INHALE** and slowly return the leg to the floor.

Repeat, then switch sides.

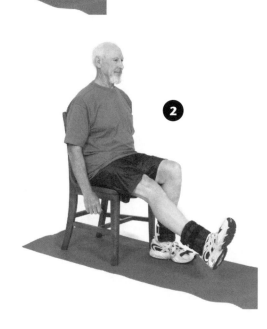

single-leg squats

target: quadriceps

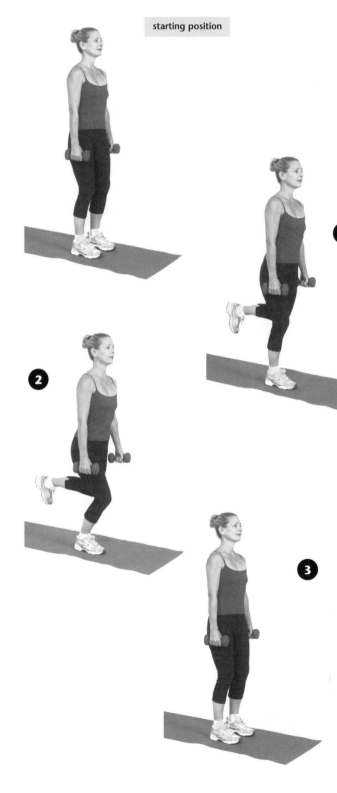

starting position

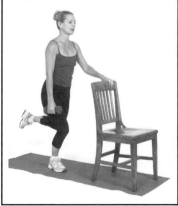

If you find this exercise too difficult, try it without weights.

STARTING POSITION: Stand with proper posture and hold a dumbbell in each hand.

1 **INHALE** and bring your left heel up halfway toward your buttocks or as high as is comfortable.

2 **EXHALE** and slowly squat down as low as you can on your other leg, keeping your foot flat on the floor.

3 **INHALE** and slowly return to full standing position.

Repeat, then switch sides.

MODIFICATION

If balance is an issue, hold one weight and hold onto a chair or wall with your free hand for support.

downhill skier

target: quadriceps

starting position

If you find this exercise too difficult, try it without weights.

STARTING POSITION: Stand with both feet as close together as is comfortable. Hold a dumbbell in each hand and cross your arms over your chest. **INHALE** to begin.

1 **EXHALE** and squat down a quarter of the way, keeping your feet flat on the floor and your knees over your toes. Do not allow your knees to turn in or out. Hold for a count of 1-2-3-4-5.

2 **INHALE** and slowly return to starting position.

1

2

MODIFICATION

If balance is an issue, try the movement without weights and hold onto a chair for support.

starting position

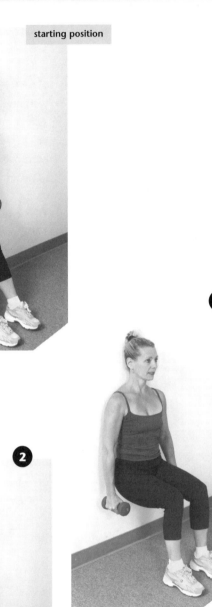

1

2

CAUTION: *If you have heart or blood-pressure issues, avoid this exercise.*

If you find this exercise too difficult, try it without weights.

STATING POSITION: Stand with your back against the wall and your feet approximately 12–18 inches from the wall. Hold a dumbbell in each hand. **INHALE** to begin.

1 Using the wall for support, **EXHALE** and lower yourself as low as is comfortable or until your thighs are parallel with the floor. Do not allow your knees to extend past your toes. Hold for a count of 1-2-3-4-5, breathing comfortably. As your strength improves, hold the position up to 30 or 60 seconds.

2 **INHALE** and slowly return to starting position.

leg curls

target: hamstrings

starting position

CAUTION: *Avoid this exercise if you have lower back issues.*

If you find this exercise too difficult, try it without weights.

STARTING POSITION: Strap an ankle weight to each ankle and stand with proper posture, both feet together. Hold on to the back of a stable chair for balance. **INHALE** to begin.

1 Slowly **EXHALE** as you curl your right leg up toward your buttocks. Stop when your leg is parallel to the ground.

2 Hold for a moment, then **INHALE** as you slowly return the leg to starting position.

Repeat, then switch sides.

1

2

prone leg curls

target: hamstrings

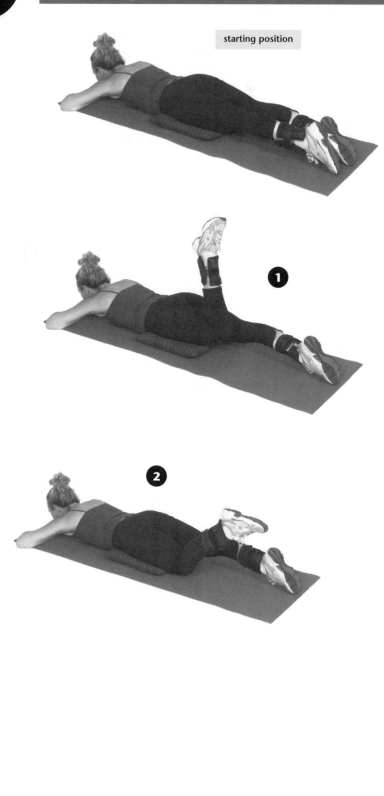

starting position

1

2

CAUTION: Avoid this exercise if lying on your stomach is uncomfortable. However, placing a pillow or rolled-up towel under your hips does help most people.

If you find this exercise too difficult, try it without weights.

STARTING POSITION: Strap an ankle weight to each ankle and lie face down on the floor. If necessary, position a pillow beneath your hips so that your back is in a comfortable neutral position. Rest your head on your forearms. **INHALE** to begin.

1 **EXHALE** and slowly bring your left heel up toward your buttock, stopping when it reaches 90 degrees.

2 **INHALE** to slowly return your foot to starting position.

Repeat, then switch sides.

VARIATION

To perform this with an exercise band, tie the ends together and loop it around both ankles.

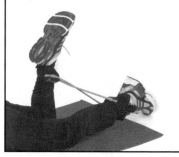

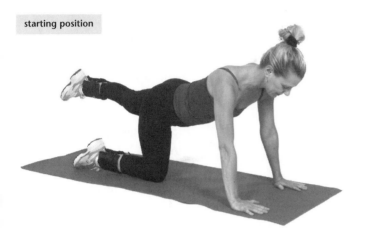

starting position

If you find this exercise too difficult, try it without weights.

STARTING POSITION: Strap an ankle weight to each ankle and get down on your hands and knees. Keeping your back straight, extend your left leg straight back and lift it up parallel to the floor; make sure your upper leg is parallel to the floor throughout the exercise. **INHALE** to begin.

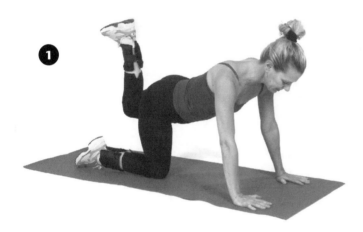

1

1 EXHALE to bend your left knee and pull your heel toward your buttocks, stopping when you reach 90 degrees. Hold for a moment. If you feel a cramp coming on, stop and stretch your leg.

2 INHALE and extend your leg back to starting position.

Repeat, then switch sides.

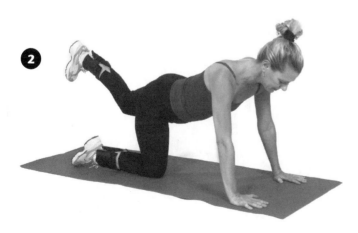

2

gas pedals

target: calves

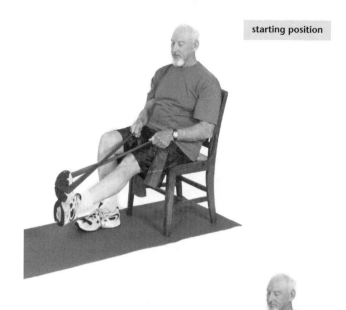

starting position

STARTING POSITION: Sit in a chair with proper posture. Extend your left leg and loop a band around your foot, crossing the band above your shin for safety. Keep your leg straight and your toes pointing straight up. **INHALE** to begin.

1 **EXHALE** and point your foot away from you, against the band's resistance. Hold for a moment.

2 **INHALE** and return to starting position.

Repeat, then switch sides.

heel raises   *target: calves*

starting position

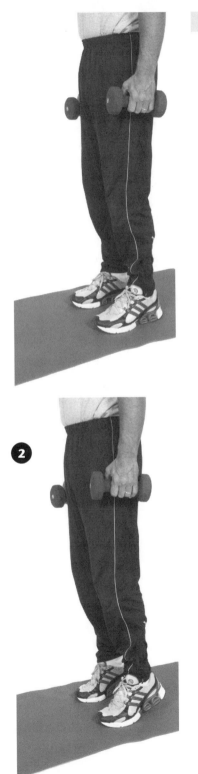

1

If you find this exercise too difficult, try it without weights.

STARTING POSITION: Stand with your feet hip-width apart and parallel to each other. Hold a dumbbell in each hand. **INHALE** to begin.

1 **EXHALE** and slowly rise up onto the balls of your feet, lifting your heels off the floor. Hold for a moment.

2 **INHALE** to slowly return to starting position.

2

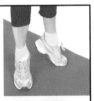

VARIATION 1

Point your toes out slightly and perform the heel raise.

VARIATION 2

Perform the move with the toes pointed slightly in.

MODIFICATION

If balance is an issue, use a chair to help steady yourself.

one-leg heel raises

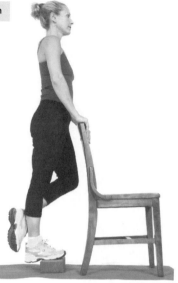

starting position

If you don't have a yoga block, you can use a 2x4 or some other solid, flat object like a telephone book.

STARTING POSITION: Place a yoga block on the floor behind a chair. Stand with the balls of your feet on the block and hold onto the chair for balance. Place your left foot behind your right heel. **INHALE** to begin.

1 EXHALE as you rise up on the ball of your right foot as high as is comfortable. Do not perform this movement to an extreme range of motion. Hold for a moment.

2 INHALE to return to starting position.

Repeat, then switch sides. Stretch your calf muscle after completing a set.

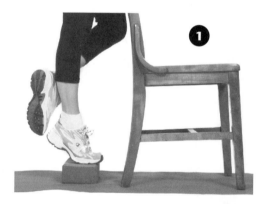

❶

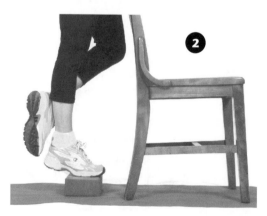

❷

curl-ups

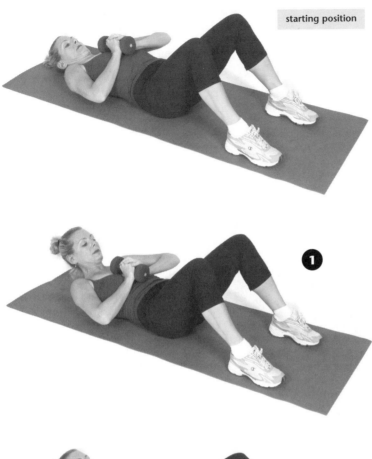

starting position

STARTING POSITION: Lie on your back with your feet flat on the floor. Hold a dumbbell in your hands on top of your chest. Tuck your chin toward your chest. **INHALE** to begin.

1 **EXHALE** as you lift your shoulders off the floor. Hold for a moment.

2 **INHALE** and slowly return to starting position.

MODIFICATION

To reduce the intensity, you can try this without weights. Place your hands lightly behind your head but be careful not to pull hard on your head.

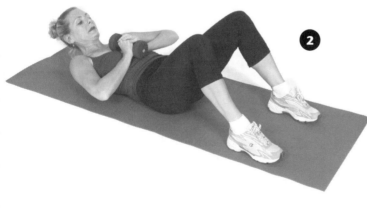

curl-ups with a twist

target: abdominals, external obliques

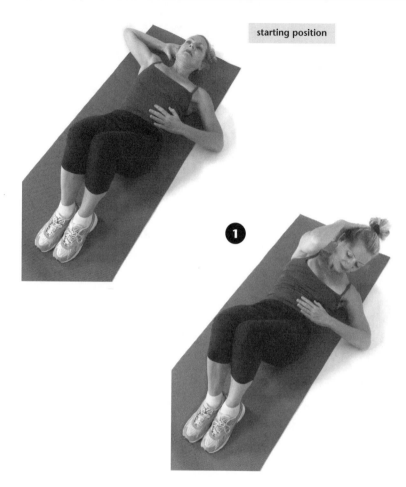

starting position

STARTING POSITION: Lie on your back with your feet flat on the floor. Place your right hand lightly behind your head. **INHALE** to begin.

1 **EXHALE** as you lift your right shoulder off the floor and gently move your right elbow toward your left knee.

2 Hold for a moment and **INHALE** as you return to starting position.

Repeat, then switch sides.

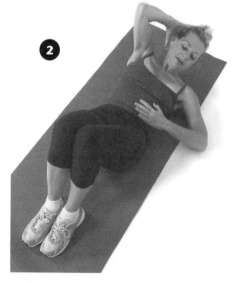

VARIATION

Lie on your back with your feet flat on the floor. Place your right ankle on your left knee, then place your left hand on your right knee. Raise your left shoulder off the floor and push your hand into your knee and your knee into your hand. Hold for 2 seconds.

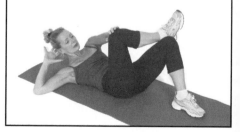

bicycle

target: abdominals

starting position

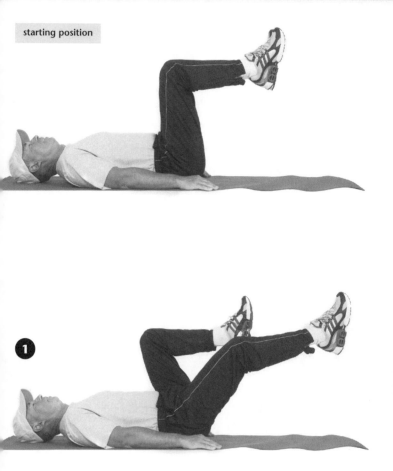

STARTING POSITION: Lie on your back with your feet flat on the floor and your arms alongside your body. Keeping your lower back neutral throughout the exercise, lift both legs off the floor as if resting them on an imaginary chair. Keep control of your core. **INHALE** to begin.

1 Without allowing your pelvis to rock or roll, **EXHALE** and contract your abdominal muscles as you press one leg forward and pull the other toward your chest.

2 **INHALE** and switch sides, pressing the other leg forward as you pull the forward leg back.

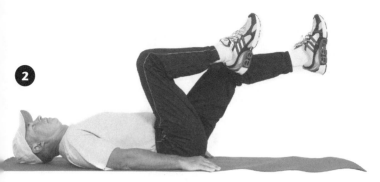

marching

starting position

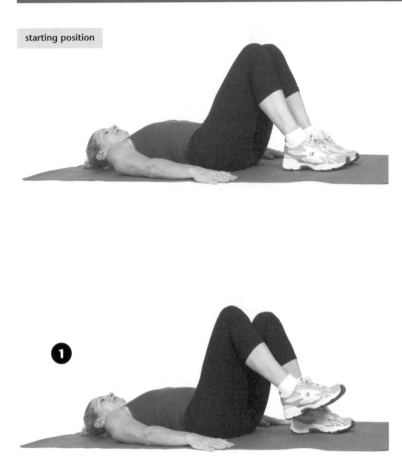

STARTING POSITION: Lie on your back with your feet flat on the floor and your arms alongside your body. Keep your core contracted and your lower back in neutral throughout the movement.

1 Imagining that a wire is pulling your knee upward, **INHALE** and slowly lift your right foot an inch or two off the floor. The smaller the distance you lift the foot off the floor (such as leaving just enough space to slip a piece of paper under), the more challenging the move.

2 **EXHALE** and slowly raise your left foot off the floor as you lower your right.

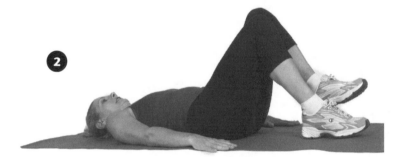

STARTING POSITION: Lie on your back with your feet flat on the floor and your arms crossed over your chest. **INHALE** to begin.

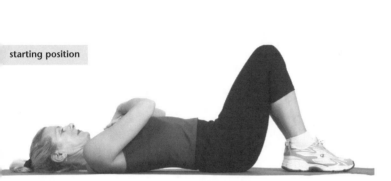

starting position

1 **EXHALE** and press your lower back into the floor (the normal curve of your spine should be lying flat so not even a piece of paper can slide between your back and the floor). Hold for a count of 1-2-3 and then relax.

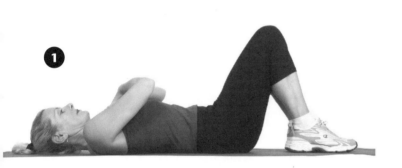

buttocks lifts

target: gluteals, back

starting position

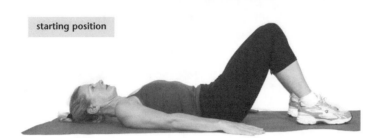

STARTING POSITION: Lie on your back with your feet flat on the floor and your arms along your sides. Press the small of your back into the floor as you tighten your core muscles. Find your neutral spine position and maintain this position throughout the exercise. **INHALE** to begin.

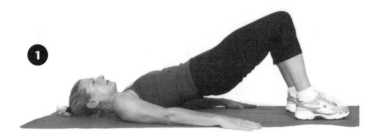

1 **EXHALE** and lift your hips and lower back off the floor. Hold this position for a moment, keeping your pelvic area stationary.

2 **INHALE** and lower yourself to the floor.

VARIATION

Perform the exercise after you've placed a band over your pelvis and secured the band in each hand at a position for ideal resistance.

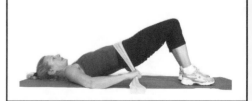

core series

pointer

starting position

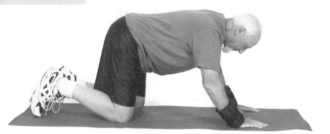

This can be very challenging. It is better to only perform a few perfectly than many with poor form. Try this without the weights if you find that they compromise your form.

STARTING POSITION: Start on your hands and knees, an ankle weight around each wrist. Pull in your abdominal muscles. Keep your back flat throughout the exercise. Breathe comfortably.

1 Lift your right arm slowly to shoulder height but no higher.

2 Return your right hand on the floor and raise your left arm.

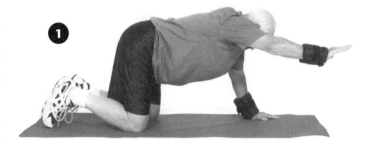

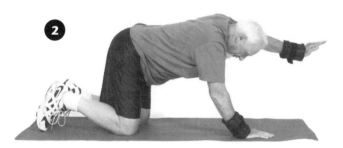

VARIATION

As your core strength improves, progress to raising your left arm and your right leg, then alternating with your right arm and your left leg. As you get stronger, you can also incorporate ankle weights.

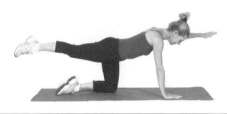

dumbbell presses

target: pectorals, front shoulders, triceps

starting position

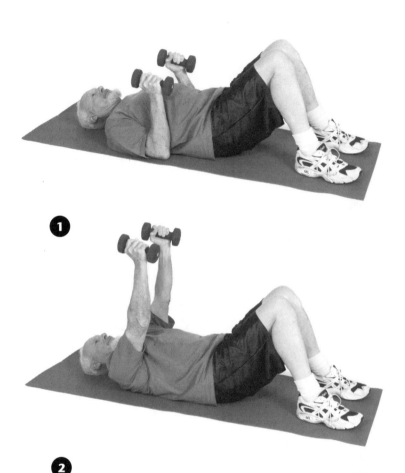

This can also be done on a sturdy bench, but do not allow your elbows to drop below your torso.

STARTING POSITION: Lie on your back with your feet flat on the floor. Hold a dumbbell in each hand with your palms facing each other, your elbows resting on the ground and your forearms perpendicular to the floor. **INHALE** to begin.

1 **EXHALE** as you slowly press the dumbbells toward the ceiling, keeping your elbows close to your sides and your arms perpendicular to the ground. Don't allow your lower back to arch, and don't lock your elbows.

2 **INHALE** as you return to starting position.

dumbbell flyes

target: pectorals

starting position

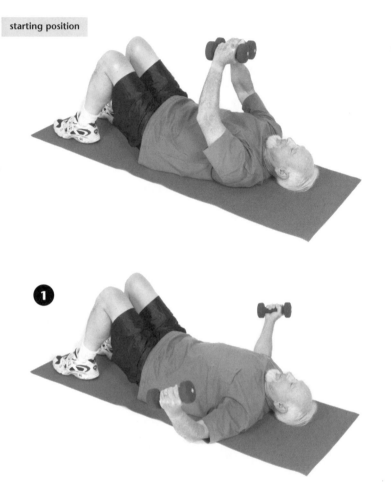

1

2

STARTING POSITION: Lie on your back with your feet flat on the floor. Hold a dumbbell in each hand with your arms extended toward the ceiling and palms facing each other. Keep your elbows slightly bent, as if you were hugging a large barrel. **INHALE** to begin.

1 **EXHALE** as you lower your arms out toward the floor to form a T; do not let your upper arms touch the ground. As you perform this move, keep your lower back flat on the floor.

2 **INHALE** as you return to starting position.

chair push-ups

target: pectorals, front shoulders, triceps

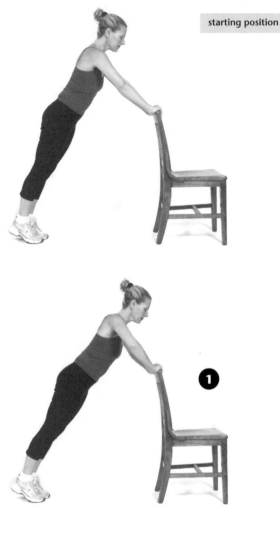

starting position

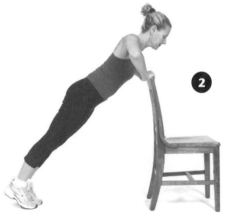

CAUTION: *Be careful not to tip over the chair.*

STARTING POSITION: Stand with proper posture next to a sturdy surface such as a chair, table or countertop. Lean forward and place your hands shoulder-width apart on the surface. Keep your arms fully extended while you walk your legs back until your body is at approximately a 45-degree angle. Your legs should be straight but not locked. **INHALE** to begin.

1 **EXHALE** as you slowly lower your chest to the chair, trying to keep your elbows close to your body. Remember to keep your torso in a straight line with your legs.

2 **INHALE** as you press your body away until your arms are fully extended without being locked.

ADVANCED VARIATION

To increase the resistance, use a sturdy surface, such as a coffee table or seat of a chair, that is closer to the ground. Once these become easy, progress to Baby Boomer Push-ups.

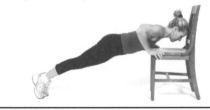

baby boomer push-ups — *target: pectorals, front shoulders, triceps*

starting position

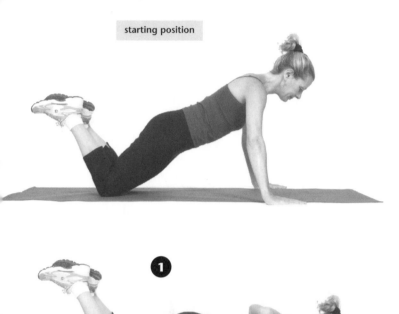

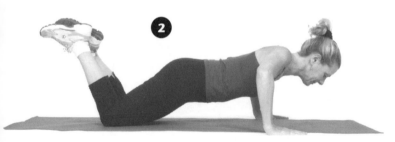

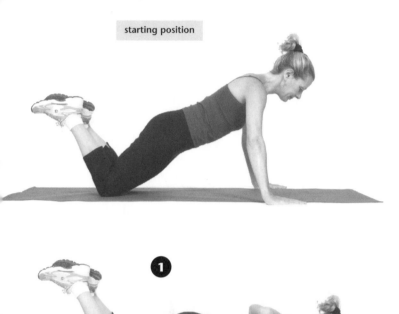

STARTING POSITION: Start on your hands and knees, moving your hands forward so that your torso is slanted yet at a comfortable angle. Keep your back straight and pull your abdominal muscles in. **INHALE** to begin.

1 EXHALE as you bend your elbows to lower your chest toward the floor. Keep your elbows close to your body and go down only as far as is comfortable. As you improve, try to get as close to the floor as possible without resting on it.

2 INHALE as you return to starting position.

ADVANCED VARIATION

As you become stronger, straighten your legs and perform the push-up from your hands and toes.

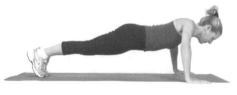

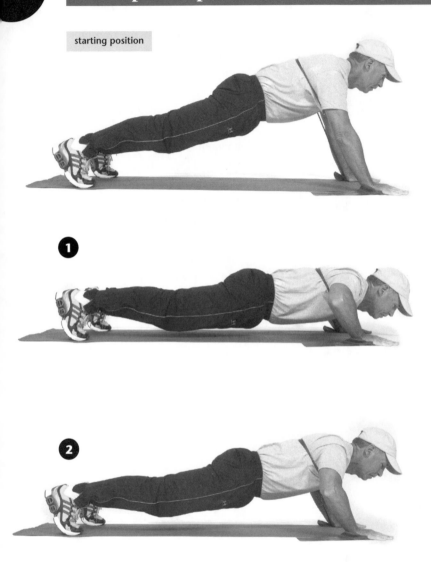

starting position

1

2

The exercise band provides additional resistance in this challenging variation of the standard push-up.

STARTING POSITION: Assume a push-up position (your body should form one plane from head to heels) and position the band around your upper back and under your arms. Keeping your arms extended, secure the ends of the bands under your hands. Spread your legs about hip-width apart. **INHALE** to begin.

1 **EXHALE** as you slowly lower your body to the floor, trying to keep your elbows close to your body. Only go as low as you feel comfortable.

2 **INHALE** as you extend your arms to starting position. Once you start to sag in the middle or lift your butt, you have lost proper form—stop!

incline presses

target: pectorals, front shoulders, triceps

starting position

STARTING POSITION: Sit with proper posture in a stable chair with your feet flat on the floor. Wrap the exercise band around your back and under your arms. Grasp the band in each hand at a length that provides adequate resistance. Position your hands close to your torso, palms facing in and elbows by your side. **INHALE** to begin.

1 **EXHALE** as you press your arms up at a 45-degree angle. Keep the movement controlled.

2 **INHALE** and resist the band as you return to starting position.

high flyes

target: pectorals, front shoulders

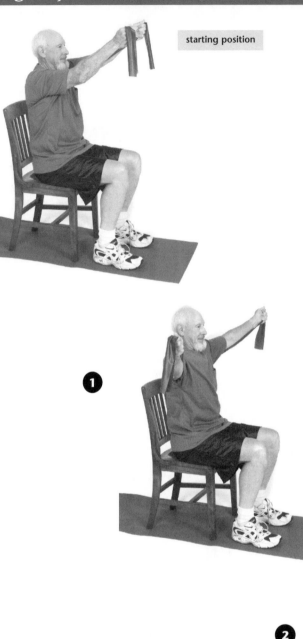

starting position

1

2

STARTING POSITION: Sit with proper posture in a stable chair with your feet flat on the floor. Wrap the exercise band around your back and under your arms. Grasp the band in each hand at a length that provides adequate resistance. Position your hands close to your torso, palms facing in and elbows by your side. Straighten your arms upward at a 45-degree angle. **INHALE** to begin.

1 **EXHALE** as you spread your arms out to the side to form a T, keeping your elbows slightly bent. Don't spread your arms so far as to hurt your shoulders. Focus on feeling the chest muscles contract.

2 **INHALE** and bring your arms back to starting position.

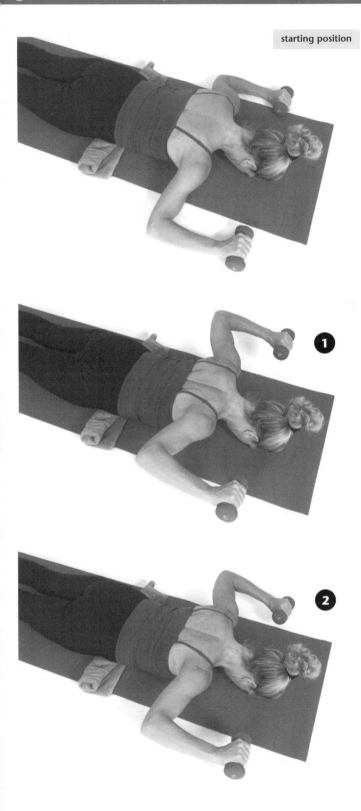

starting position

1

2

CAUTION: Do not perform this move if you have lower back issues—do Reverse Band Flyes instead.

This exercise can also be done on a sturdy bench or weight bench, but do not do so if you have poor balance.

STARTING POSITION: Lie face down on the ground, keeping your head in line with your spine. Position a rolled-up towel under your hips so that your back is comfortable. Grasp a dumbbell in each hand and position your legs to provide the most support and balance possible.

1 **INHALE** and, while squeezing your shoulder blades together, slowly lift your arms toward the ceiling until they are parallel to the ground. Do not lift your arms higher than your shoulders.

2 **EXHALE** and slowly lower your arms to starting position.

single-arm rows

target: upper back, rear shoulders

starting position

CAUTION: *Do not do this exercise if you have back issues.*

STARTING POSITION: Stand behind a stable chair and place your left hand on the chair's back. Position your left leg forward and right leg back a comfortable distance apart, keeping your knees slightly bent and upper body angled forward. Grasp a dumbbell in your right hand with your elbow slightly bent, as if you are about to start a lawnmower. Tighten your core muscles to protect your back. **INHALE** to begin.

1 **EXHALE** as you slowly pull your right hand in toward your right armpit, pinching your shoulder blades together. Do not twist your torso.

2 **INHALE** and slowly return to starting position.

Repeat, then switch sides.

1

2

starting position

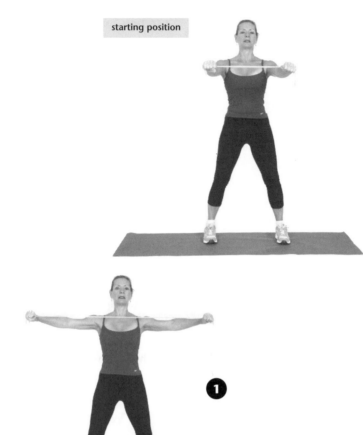

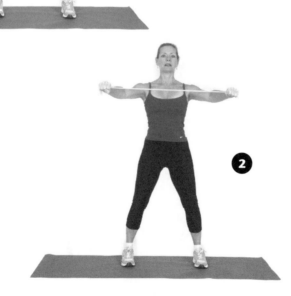

CAUTION: If you feel discomfort in your shoulders, STOP!

This can be done while standing or sitting.

STARTING POSITION: Stand with proper posture. Hold an exercise band in front of you with your palms facing down, shoulder-width apart. Grasp the band at a place that provides adequate resistance. Raise your arms to shoulder height, keeping them straight but not locked. **INHALE** to begin.

1 **EXHALE** and slowly spread your arms to the side. Only go as far apart as you can still see your hands. Don't allow your shoulders to shrug and don't arch your back.

2 **INHALE** and slowly return to starting position.

pull-downs

target: upper back

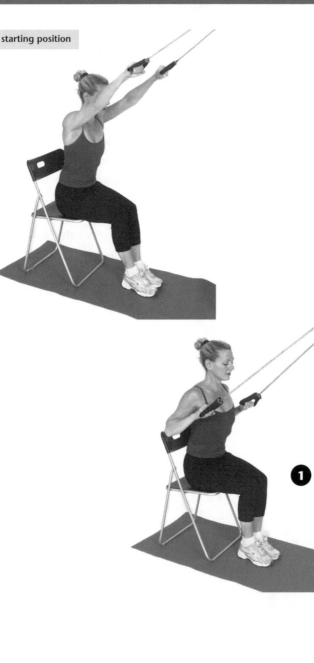

starting position

STARTING POSITION: Attach an exercise band to a solid overhead item (loops are available at sporting goods stores). Sit in a chair and lean slightly forward toward the band's attachment. Reach up and grasp the band at a place that provides adequate resistance. Keep your torso firm to protect your back. **INHALE** to begin.

1 **EXHALE** and, while squeezing your shoulder blades together, slowly pull your hands down toward your shoulders.

2 **INHALE** and return slowly to the starting position.

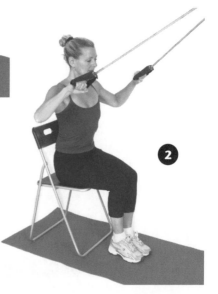

y pull-downs

target: upper back

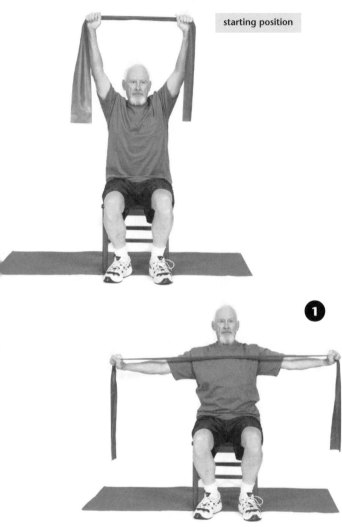

starting position

①

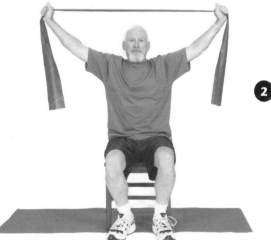

②

This exercise can be done while standing or sitting. You can also alternate arms.

STARTING POSITION: Sit in a chair with proper posture. With your palms forward, shoulder-width apart, grasp an end of the band in each hand at a place that provides adequate resistance. Raise your arms overhead. **INHALE** to begin.

1 **EXHALE** and slowly lower your arms to the sides, stopping at shoulder level. Don't arch your back.

2 **INHALE** and return to starting position.

shoulder retractions

target: upper back, rear shoulders

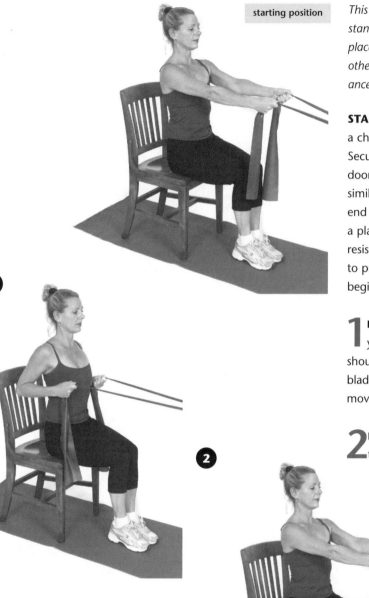

starting position

This exercise can be done while standing or sitting. If standing, place one leg forward and the other back for support and balance. You can also alternate arms.

STARTING POSITION: Sit in a chair with proper posture. Securely attach a band to the doorknob of a closed door or similar stable object. Grasp an end of the band in each hand at a place that provides adequate resistance. Keep your core firm to protect your back. **INHALE** to begin.

1 **EXHALE** as you slowly pull your hands toward your shoulders. Keep your shoulder blades together at all times, moving only your arms.

2 **INHALE** as you slowly return to starting position.

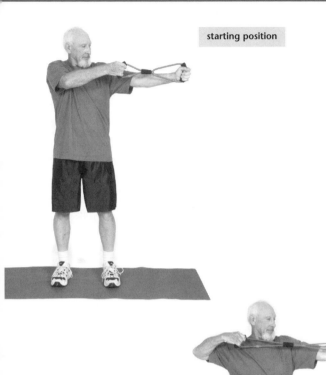

starting position

This exercise can be done while standing or sitting.

STARTING POSITION: Stand with proper posture. Grasp one end of the band with your left hand, then extend the arm out to the side at shoulder height. With your right hand, reach across your body and grasp the band near your left elbow.

1 **INHALE** as you pull the band across your chest toward your right shoulder, as if pulling a bow.

2 **EXHALE** as you return to starting position.

Repeat, then switch sides.

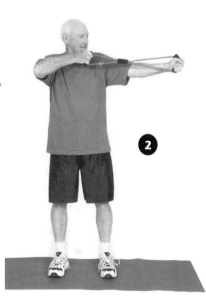

seated rows

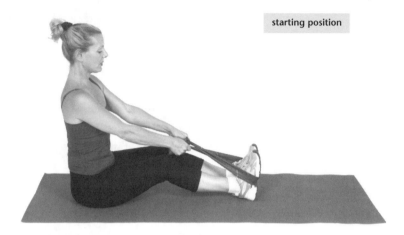

starting position

This exercise can also be done while sitting in a chair.

STARTING POSITION: Sit on the floor and extend your legs out in front of you. Loop an exercise band around your feet, crossing the band over your shins to provide better safety. With your palms facing each other, grasp the band at a position for ideal resistance. **INHALE** to begin.

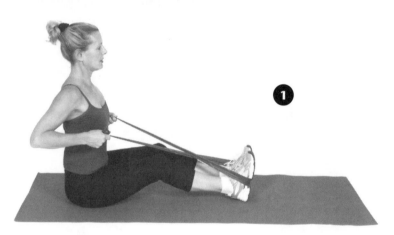

1 **EXHALE** as you slowly pull your hands toward your chest, trying to keep your arms close to your body. Focus on keeping your shoulder blades together throughout the movement and only move your arms.

2 **INHALE** as you slowly return to starting position.

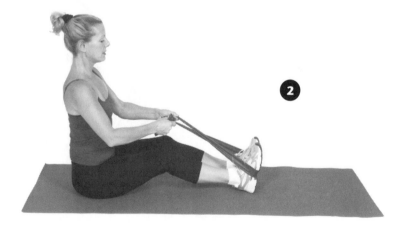

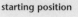
starting position

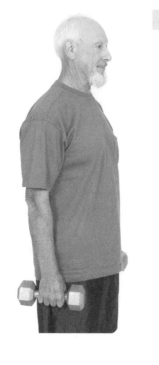

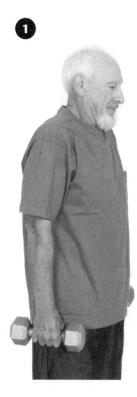

1

2

STARTING POSITION: Stand with proper posture and hold a dumbbell in each hand. Extend your arms straight alongside your body.

1 **INHALE** as you slowly "shrug" your shoulders up toward your ears.

2 **EXHALE** and roll your shoulders back, slowly lowering your shoulders to starting position.

lateral arm raises

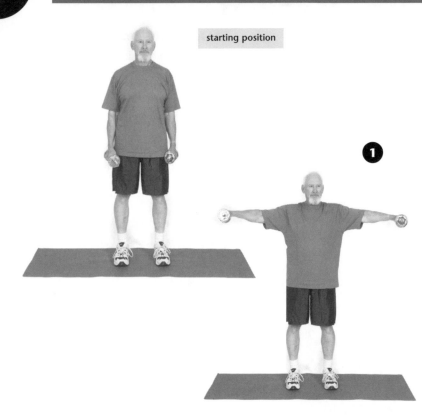

starting position

①

CAUTION: If you feel clicking in the shoulder area while doing this exercise, STOP!

If you feel any discomfort in your lower back, re-adjust your posture and try the exercise by alternating your arms.

STARTING POSITION: Stand with proper posture with your arms straight alongside your body and hold a dumbbell in each hand. Keep your torso firm to protect your lower back.

1 **INHALE** as you slowly lift your arms out to the side, no higher than shoulder level.

2 **EXHALE** as you slowly return to starting position.

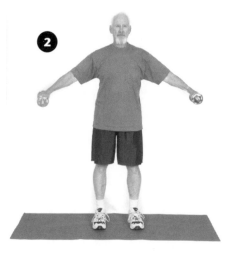

②

VARIATION

Stand on the exercise band and with both hands grasp the band at a position that provides adequate resistance.

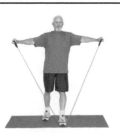

MODIFICATIONS

If doing this exercise with straight arms is too difficult, flare your elbows out like a chicken.

If your arms feel uncomfortable going out to the side, try moving them slightly forward to see if the motion feels better.

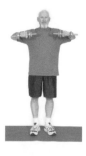

frontal arm raises

target: front shoulders, upper back

starting position

If you feel any discomfort in your lower back, re-adjust your posture and don't go as high.

STARTING POSITION: Stand with proper posture. Hold a dumbbell in each hand with your arms straight, but not locked, and your palms facing your thighs. Keep your torso firm to protect your lower back.

1 **INHALE** and slowly raise your right arm forward to shoulder height but no higher.

1

2 **EXHALE** as you lower your arm to the starting position more slowly than when you lifted it. Alternate arms.

2

VARIATION

Stand on one end of the exercise band then grasp the band at a position that provides adequate resistance.

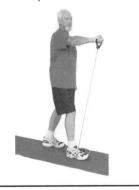

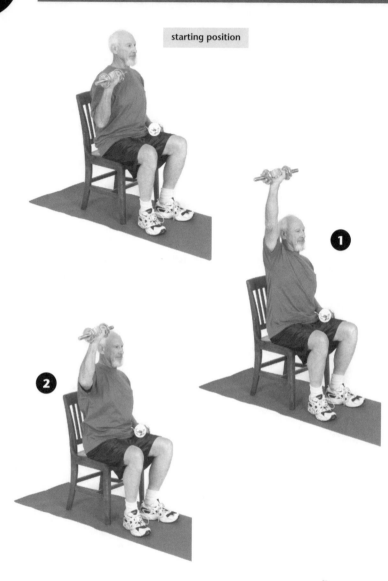

starting position

1

2

CAUTION: *Avoid this exercise if you have a history of shoulder or lower back complaints or have osteoporosis/osteopenia.*

This exercise can be done while standing or sitting. If done from a standing position, don't arch your back—maintain proper neutral spine at all times.

STARTING POSITION: Sit with proper posture on a stable chair. Hold a dumbbell in your right hand next to your right shoulder with your palm facing forward. Make sure you are balanced and keep your back in its neutral position. **INHALE** to begin.

1 **EXHALE** as you press your right arm to the ceiling. Your arm doesn't need to extend directly above your shoulder— slightly forward is acceptable.

2 **INHALE** as you lower the dumbbell slowly to starting position.

Repeat then switch sides.

VARIATION 1

Wrap an exercise band around your back and under your arms. Hold an end of the band in each hand, adjusting the band length to regulate the resistance.

VARIATION 2

Try positioning your palms inward and perform the same movement. See which feels most comfortable to you.

upright rows

target: shoulders, upper back, biceps

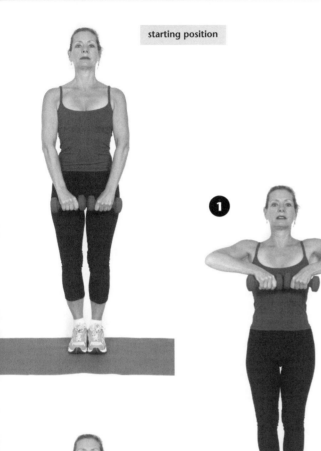

starting position

1

2

CAUTION: If you have a history of shoulder problems, avoid this exercise.

STARTING POSITION: Stand with proper posture. Hold a dumbbell in each hand with your arms in front of your body and your palms facing your thighs. **INHALE** to begin.

1 Keeping your hands close to your body, bend your elbows and **EXHALE** as you pull the dumbbells up to chest level. Don't allow your wrists to go higher than your elbows or your elbows to go higher than your shoulders, and don't arch your back.

2 **INHALE** as you slowly lower the dumbbells to starting position, resisting the force of gravity by keeping your muscles tense.

MODIFICATION

If your shoulders feel uncomfortable, try pulling the dumbbells up alongside your body until they reach your armpits. If you still feel discomfort, avoid this exercise.

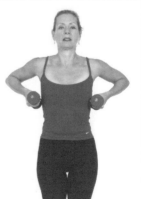

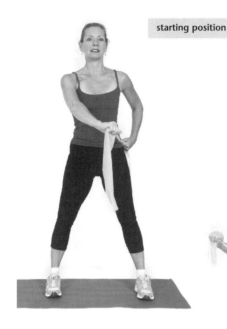

starting position

This can also be done while sitting.

STARTING POSITION: Stand with proper posture. Hold an end of the band on your left hip with your left hand then grasp the band with your right hand, thumb down, at the point that will provide adequate resistance. Keep your right arm straight but not locked. **INHALE** to begin.

1 **EXHALE** as you slowly pull the band diagonally across your body as if pulling out a sword.

2 **INHALE** as you return to starting position.

Repeat, then switch sides.

1

2

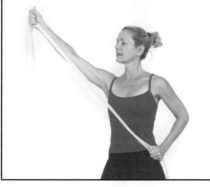

VARIATION
Grab the band with your thumb up to activate the front deltoid.

reverse sword fighter

target: rear shoulders, upper back

starting position

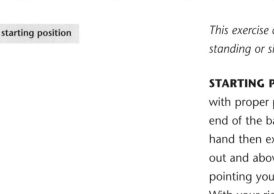

This exercise can be done while standing or sitting.

STARTING POSITION: Stand with proper posture. Hold an end of the band in your left hand then extend your left arm out and above your left shoulder, pointing your thumb down. With your right hand, thumb up, grasp the other end of the band at a point that provides adequate resistance. Keep your left arm stationary. **INHALE** to begin.

1 **EXHALE** and slowly pull the right arm down alongside the right side of your body.

2 **INHALE** as you return to starting position.

Repeat, then switch sides.

internal rotations

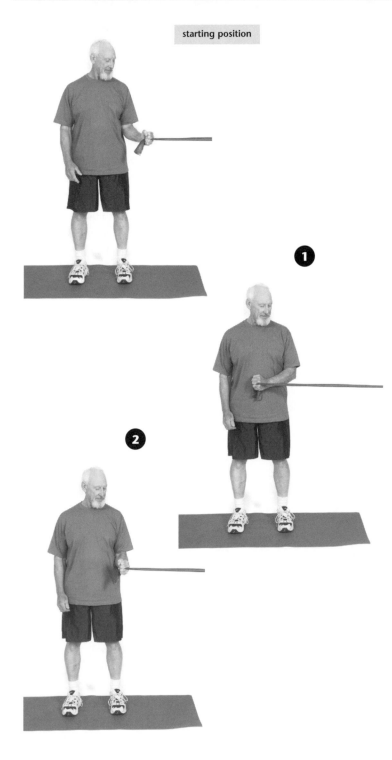

starting position

CAUTION: *Do not perform this exercise quickly as you may harm yourself.*

You can also use a doorknob instead of a chair (door attachment devices are commercially available). To reinforce proper positioning, you may want to place a towel between your elbow and torso.

STARTING POSITION: Attach the band securely to a stable chair so that you'll be pulling the band at belly button height. Stand with the left side of your body next to the chair. Grasp the band with your left hand, thumb up and palm facing in. Bend your right elbow 90 degrees and keep it close to your body. Stay mindful of engaging the deep muscles of the shoulder area. **INHALE** to begin.

1 Moving only your forearm, **EXHALE** as you slowly bring your right hand toward your belly button.

2 **INHALE** as you slowly return to starting position.

Repeat, then switch sides.

external rotations
target: rotator cuff

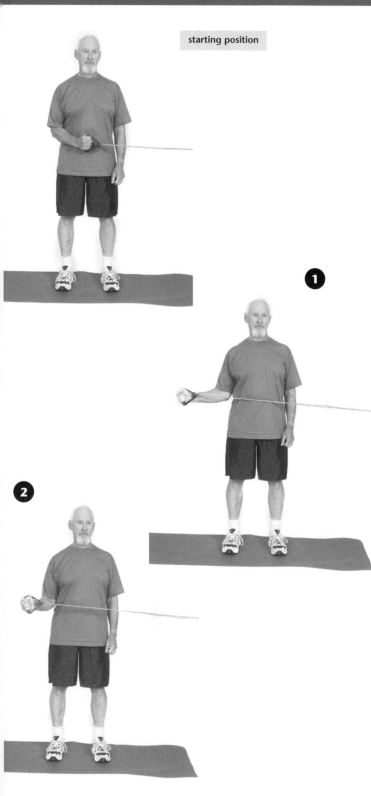

starting position

1

2

CAUTION: *Do not perform this exercise quickly as you may harm yourself.*

You can also use a doorknob instead of a chair (door attachment devices are commercially available).

STARTING POSITION: Attach the band securely to a sturdy chair so that you'll be pulling the band at belly button height. Stand with the left side of your body a band's distance away from the chair. Reach across your body to grasp the band with your right hand, thumb facing up. Bend your right elbow 90 degrees and keep it next to your body. Stay mindful of engaging the deep muscles of the shoulder area. Resistance is not important in this exercise. **INHALE** to begin.

1 With your right elbow next to your body and moving only your lower arm, **EXHALE** and slowly move your right hand away from your body, leading with your knuckles. Do not twist your torso.

2 **INHALE** and slowly return to starting position.

Repeat, then switch sides.

biceps curls

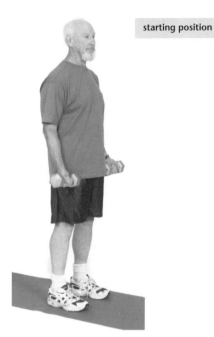

starting position

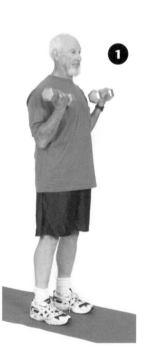

1

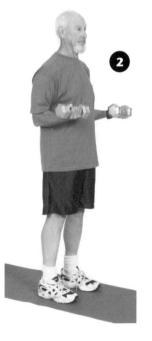

2

These curls can be done using both arms simultaneously or alternately; they can also be done while standing or sitting.

STARTING POSITION: Stand with proper posture, feet hip-width apart. Hold a dumbbell in each hand with your palms facing up, keeping your elbows tucked against your torso. Keep your torso firm to protect your lower back. **INHALE** to begin.

1 **EXHALE** as you slowly curl the dumbbells toward your shoulders.

2 **INHALE** and slowly lower your arms to starting position.

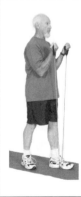

VARIATION

Place your left foot in the center of the band and grasp the ends in each hand at a place that allows the band to be taut and provide adequate resistance. (To increase the workload, grab lower on the band.) Keep your torso firm and your elbows close to your body. Perform the curl from here.

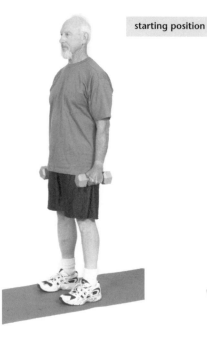

starting position

These curls can be done using both arms simultaneously or alternately; they can also be done while standing or sitting.

STARTING POSITION: Stand with proper posture, feet hip-width apart. Hold a dumbbell in each hand with your thumbs forward, keeping your elbows tucked against your torso. Keep your torso firm to protect your lower back. **INHALE** to begin.

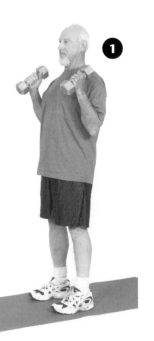

1 **EXHALE** as you slowly curl the dumbbells toward your shoulders.

2 **INHALE** and slowly lower your arms to starting position.

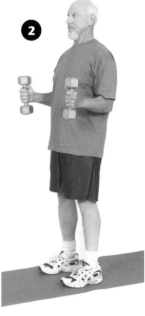

VARIATION

Place your left foot on the center of the band and grasp the ends with your left hand at a place that allows the band to be taut and provide adequate resistance. (To increase the workload, grab lower on the band.) Keep your torso firm and your elbow close to your body. Perform the curl from here.

cross-your-heart curls

starting position

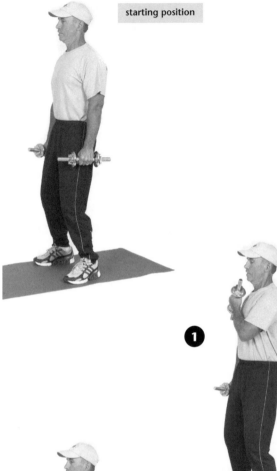

These curls can be done using both arms simultaneously or alternately; they can also be done while standing or sitting.

STARTING POSITION: Stand with proper posture, feet hip-width apart. Hold a dumbbell in each hand with your palms facing your legs, keeping your elbows tucked against your torso. Keep your torso firm to protect your lower back. **INHALE** to begin.

1 **EXHALE** as you slowly curl your hand across your body to take your left hand to your right shoulder.

2 **INHALE** and slowly lower your left arm to starting position. Now **EXHALE** and slowly curl your right hand to your left shoulder. **INHALE** and return to starting position.

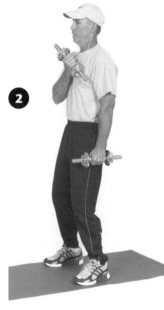

concentration curls

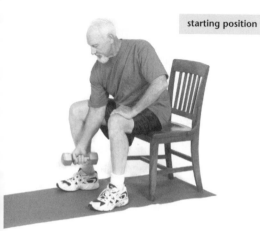

starting position

STARTING POSITION: Sit at the end of a bench or chair and lean slightly forward. Place your left hand on your left thigh for support and place your right elbow on the inside of your right thigh. Grasp a dumbbell with your right hand, palm up. Start with your arm straight but not locked and keep your elbow pressed against your thigh. **INHALE** to begin.

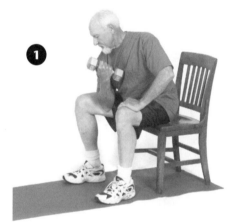

1 **EXHALE** and curl your right hand toward your right shoulder.

2 **INHALE** and slowly return to starting position.

Repeat, then switch arms.

VARIATION

You can also grasp the dumbbell with your thumb up.

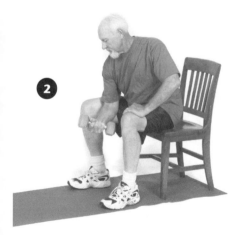

reverse curls

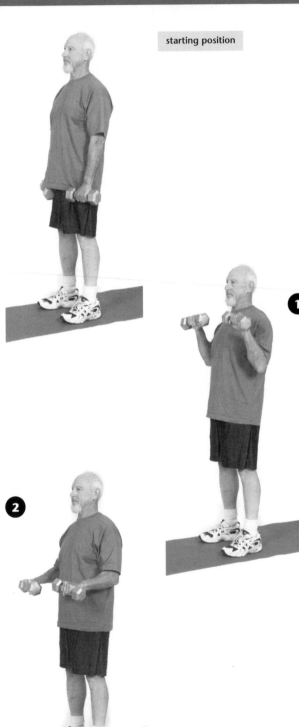

starting position

These curls can be done using both arms simultaneously or alternately; they can also be done while standing or sitting.

STARTING POSITION: Stand with proper posture, feet hip-width apart. Hold a dumbbell in each hand, with your knuckles facing forward. Keep your elbows tucked against your torso. **INHALE** to begin.

1 **EXHALE** as you slowly curl your arms up, bringing your knuckles toward your shoulders.

2 **INHALE** as you slowly lower your arms to starting position.

wrist curls

starting position

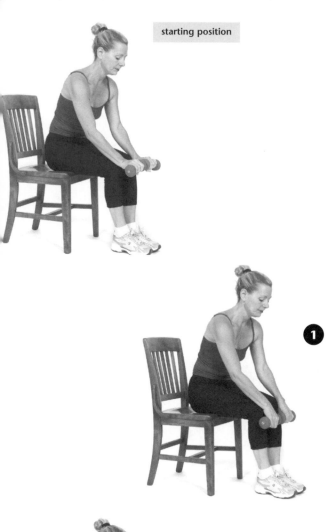

CAUTION: If you have arthritis of the wrist, consult your doctor before doing this.

Keep the weights light and work up to higher repetitions. You can also do this exercise one arm at a time.

STARTING POSITION: Sit in a stable chair. Hold a dumbbell in each hand and rest your forearms on your thighs so that your hands extend over your knees. Breathe in a comfortable manner.

1 Allow your wrists to (flex) relax downward.

2 Slowly bring your knuckles upward to return to starting position.

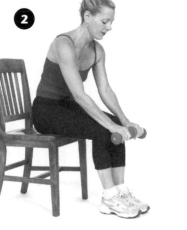

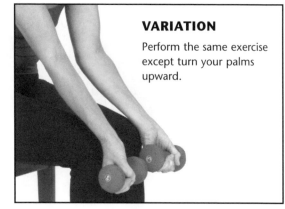

VARIATION

Perform the same exercise except turn your palms upward.

side-lying triceps extensions

starting position

STARTING POSITION: Lie on the left side of your body in a comfortable and stable position. Hold a dumbbell in your right hand close to your right shoulder, with your elbow up and your thumb down. **INHALE** to begin.

1 **EXHALE** and, hinging slowly from your elbow, extend your right hand up toward the ceiling.

2 **INHALE** and slowly return to starting position.

Repeat, then switch sides.

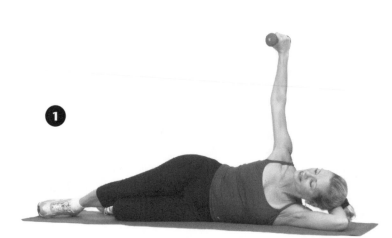

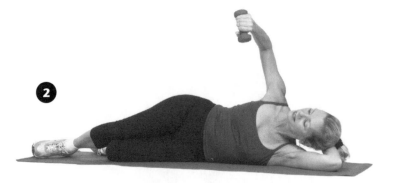

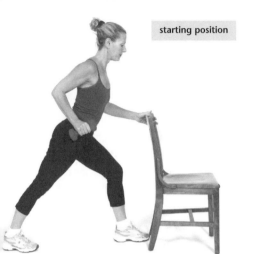

starting position

STARTING POSITION: Standing with one foot in front of the other for stability, bend over at the waist and rest your left hand on a chair. Grasp a dumbbell in your right hand, keeping your right elbow close to your torso so that your upper arm is at a 45-degree angle with the floor. **INHALE** to begin.

1 **EXHALE**, keeping your right upper arm stationary and at a 45-degree angle with the floor, as you slowly extend your arm at the elbow to full extension, but avoid locking your elbow and don't let your arm swing up.

2 **INHALE** as you return to starting position.

Repeat, then switch sides.

supine triceps extensions

starting position

CAUTION: *If you feel any discomfort in your elbow or shoulder, stop.*

This exercise can be performed by alternating arms or using them simultaneously.

STARTING POSITION: Lie on your back with your feet flat on the floor. Hold a dumbbell in each hand with your palms facing each other and your arms extended above your shoulders. **INHALE** to begin.

1

1 EXHALE and, hinging only at the elbows, lower the dumbbells toward your shoulders, stopping when your elbows make 90-degree angles. Keep your elbows pointed toward the ceiling.

2

2 INHALE as you slowly return to starting position.

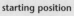
starting position

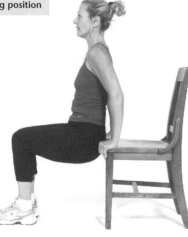

CAUTION: Be careful the chair does not tip over.

You can also do this on a counter-top or a coffee table.

STARTING POSITION: Sit in a solid and stable chair. Place your hands flat on the seat, fingers pointing toward the edge, and slide forward until your bottom is just off the seat. **INHALE** to begin.

1 **EXHALE** as you slowly bend your elbows, trying to keep them close to your torso as you lower your bottom toward the floor.

2 **INHALE** as you return to starting position.

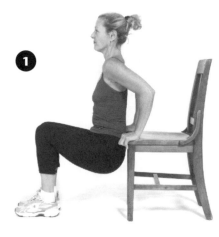

1

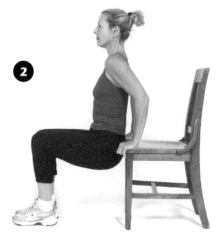

2

ADVANCED VARIATION

As you get stronger, extend your legs out farther from the chair.

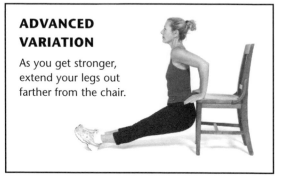

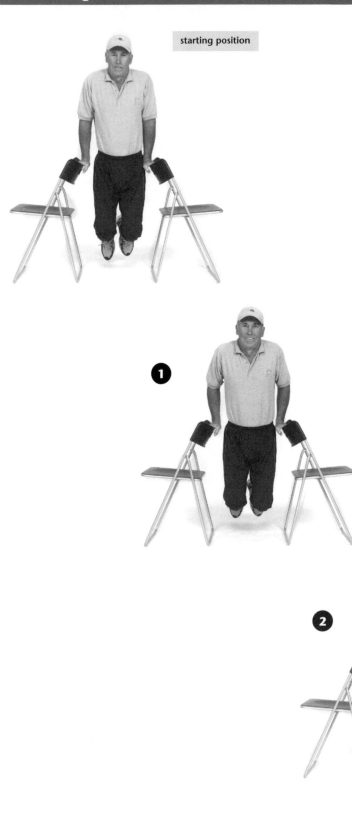

starting position

1

2

CAUTION: *Be careful the chairs do not tip over.*

This is a challenging move. If needed, rest your feet lightly on the floor behind you.

STARTING POSITION: Position two sturdy chairs with their backs parallel to each other. Space them apart so that you can stand between them and place your hands on the tops.

1 **INHALE** as you slowly bend your elbows and lower your bottom toward the floor.

2 **EXHALE** as you return to starting position.

triceps band extensions

target: triceps

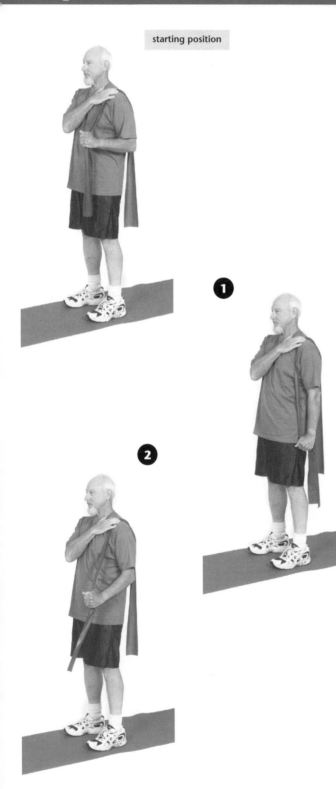

starting position

STARTING POSITION: Stand with proper posture and drape the exercise band over your left shoulder and place your right hand on your left shoulder to secure it. Keep your left elbow next to your body and grasp the band with your left hand to make a 90-degree angle with your arm; make sure the band is taut at all times. Keep your right and left hand lined up. **INHALE** to begin.

1 Without using momentum, **EXHALE** as you slowly extend your left arm downward.

2 **INHALE** and even more slowly return to starting position.

Repeat, then switch sides.

horizontal triceps extensions

starting position

This can also be done with both arms simultaneously, or while sitting.

STARTING POSITION: Stand with proper posture and grasp the band with both hands, palms down. The closer you position your hands toward the middle of the band, the more resistance you will have. Lift your elbows up and away from your body so that everything is at shoulder height. Keep your torso firm to protect your lower back. **INHALE** to begin.

1 **EXHALE** as you slowly extend your right arm out to the side.

2 **INHALE** and return to starting position even more slowly.

3 Alternate sides.

1

2

soup can pours

target: shoulders, rotator cuff

STARTING POSITION: Stand with proper posture, your arms at your side and your palms facing back.

1 **INHALE** deeply through your nose and bring both arms slightly forward as your raise them out to the sides, keeping your palm facing back. Raise your arms no higher than shoulder level.

2 **EXHALE** as you lower your arms.

starting position

elbow touches

target: chest, shoulders

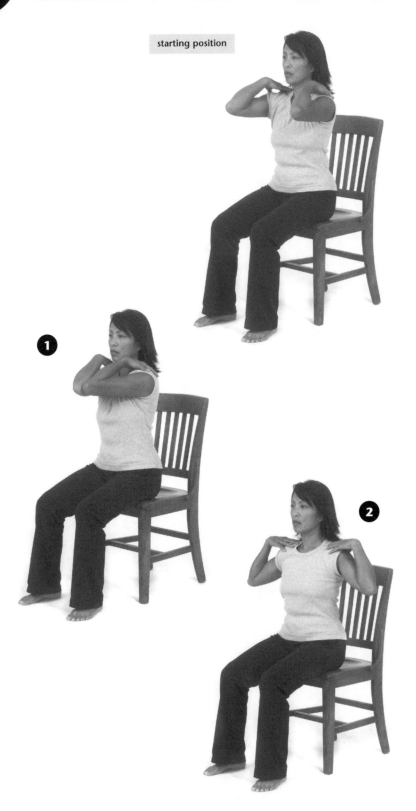

starting position

1

2

You can also try this stretch standing with proper posture.

STARTING POSITION: Sit with proper posture in a stable chair. Place your hands on your shoulders.

1 Slowly bring your elbows together in front of your body.

2 Bring your elbows back and squeeze your shoulder blades together. Hold for a moment, focusing on opening up your chest.

Bring your elbows back to the starting position and repeat as desired.

VARIATION
Once you've done Step 2, draw circles with your elbows.

stretches

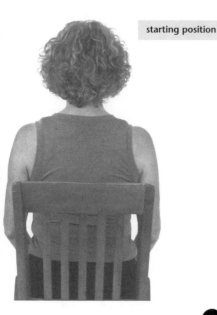

starting position

You can also try this stretch standing with proper posture.

STARTING POSITION: Sit with proper posture in a stable chair.

1 Raise your right arm and place your hand on your back, over your right shoulder.

2 Place your left hand on your right elbow and gently press your right arm down your back as far as feels comfortable. Hold the position for a comfortable moment.

Switch sides and repeat.

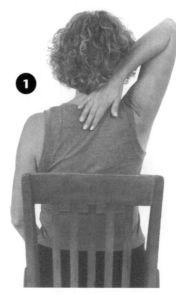

1

2

VARIATION

In Step 2, press your right arm down as you push your right elbow up into your hand. Hold this position for a comfortable moment, remembering to breathe. Then release and allow your hand to slide a little further down your back.

choker

target: shoulders, rotator cuff

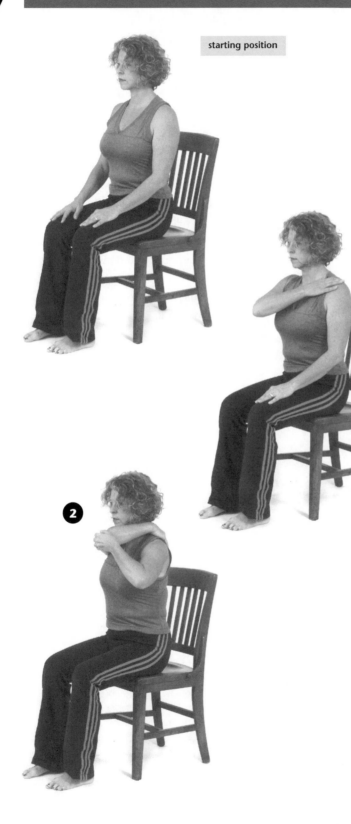

starting position

①

②

You can also try this stretch standing with proper posture.

STARTING POSITION: Sit with proper posture in a stable chair.

1 Place your right hand on your left shoulder.

2 Place your left hand on your right elbow and gently press your right elbow toward your throat. Hold for a comfortable moment.

Switch sides and repeat.

VARIATION

In Step 2, press your right elbow into your left hand. Hold for a comfortable moment, remembering to breathe. Then release to reach the right hand a little farther back.

starting position

You can also try this stretch standing with proper posture.

STARTING POSITION: Sit with proper posture in a stable chair. Place your hands behind your head.

1 Gently move your elbows back and try to bring your shoulder blades together. Focus on opening up the chest and tightening the upper back muscles. Only go as far back as is comfortable and hold for a moment.

Repeat as desired.

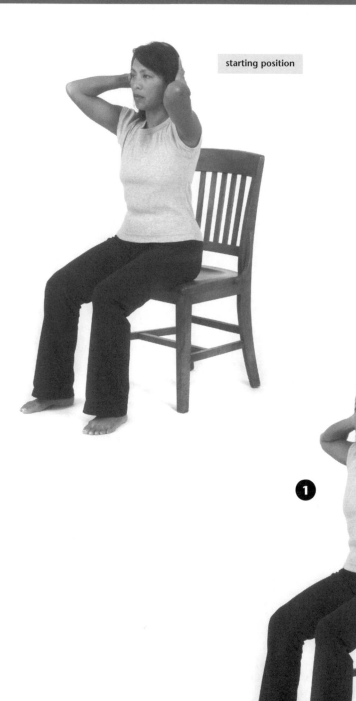

1

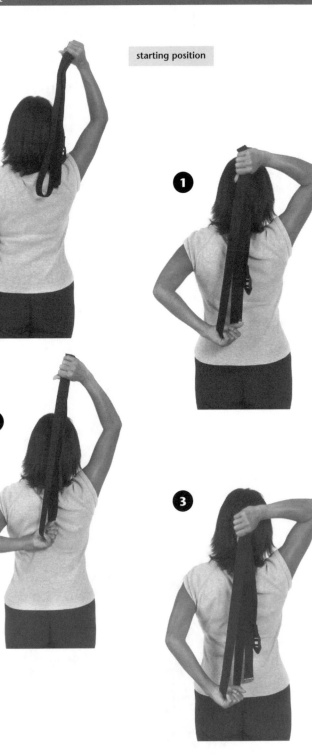

starting position

1

2

3

You can also try this stretch standing with proper posture.

STARTING POSITION: Stand with proper posture. Hold a strap in your right hand and raise your arm above your head.

1 Bring your right hand down behind your head and grab the dangling end of the strap with your lower hand.

2 Raise your right hand up as high as possible to lift the lower hand, staying in your pain-free zone. Hold the position for a comfortable moment.

3 Pull down with the lower hand to bring down the higher hand. Hold the position for a comfortable moment.

Switch sides and repeat.

ADVANCED

As you become more flexible, eliminate the use of the strap and try to grab your fingertips.

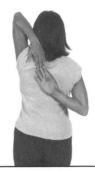

seated knee to chest   *target: lower back, gluteus maximus*

starting position

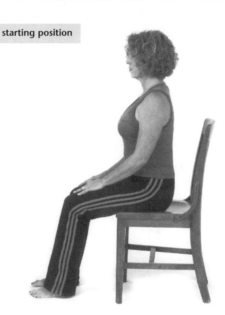

STARTING POSITION: Sit with proper posture in a stable chair and place your feet on the floor.

1 Clasp both hands beneath your left leg.

2 Bring your left knee toward your chest. Hold this position for a comfortable moment, feeling the stretch in the gluteal region.

Release the knee, switch sides and repeat.

1

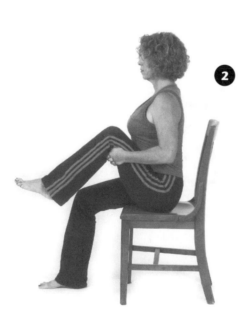

2

double knee to chest

target: lower back, gluteus maximus

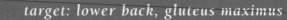

starting position

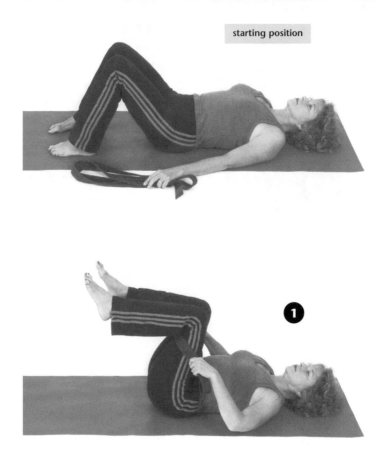

1

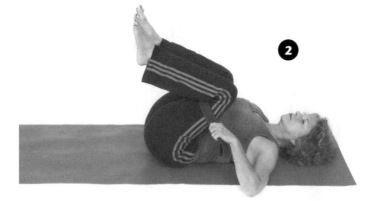

2

STARTING POSITION: Lie on a mat and, if needed, place a pillow under your head. Bend your knees and place both feet flat on the floor.

1 Loop a strap behind the backs of both legs and hold an end of the strap in each hand.

2 Gently pull the straps to bring your knees to your chest. Hold this position for a comfortable moment, feeling the stretch in your bottom and low back.

ADVANCED

Use just your hands to draw in your knees.

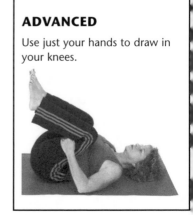

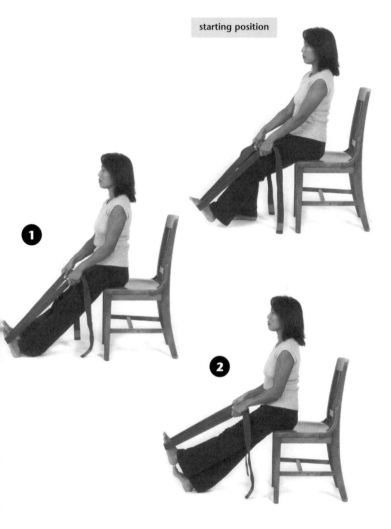

starting position

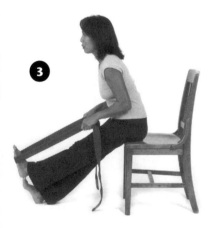

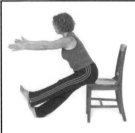

CAUTION: *Be careful not to tip the chair over.*

STARTING POSITION: Sit at the edge of a stable chair. Loop a strap around the ball of your left foot and hold an end of the strap in each hand.

1 Extend your legs straight out in front of you and place your heels on the floor with your toes pointing up close to 90 degrees.

2 Stack your left heel on top of your right foot, keeping your legs as straight as possible. Inhale deeply through your nose.

3 Now exhale through your lips and gently pull yourself forward by leading with your chest rather than rounding your back.

Switch sides and repeat.

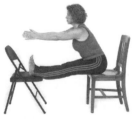

INTERMEDIATE

Instead of using the strap, you can extend your arms forward and gently reach forward with your fingertips.

ADVANCED

Place both heels on a chair in front of you.

starting position

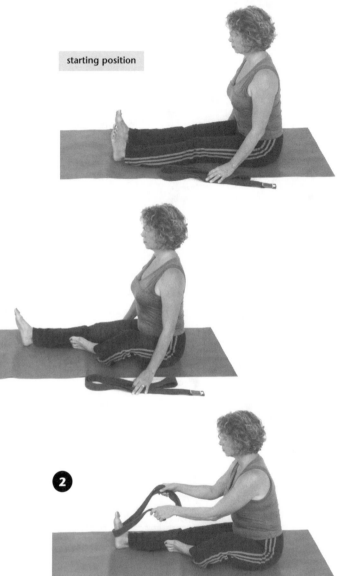

CAUTION: *Avoid this move if you have knee problems.*

STARTING POSITION: Sit on a mat with both legs extended straight out in front of you. Keep your torso as tall as possible.

1 Place your left foot against your right knee.

2 Loop a strap around the sole of your right foot and hold on to the ends of the strap. Inhale deeply through your nose.

3 While keeping your head and torso tall, pull yourself forward until you feel a comfortable stretch in the backs of your legs. Hold this stretch for a comfortable moment, focusing on the sensation of the stretch, not on going as far as possible. The goal is to hold the stretch for 60 seconds. Exhale through your lips and return to the starting position.

Switch sides and repeat.

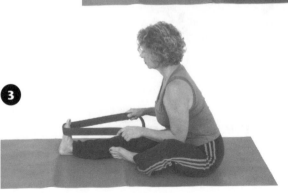

rear calf stretch

starting position

STARTING POSITION: Stand behind a chair, placing both hands on the back of the chair.

1 Keeping the heel down, slide your right leg as far back as you can.

2 Bend your left knee until the desired stretch is felt in the calf area. Hold this stretch for a comfortable moment.

Switch sides and repeat.

1

2

index

about the author

KARL KNOPF, author of *Stretching for 50+* (Ulysses Press), has been involved with the health and fitness of the disabled and older adults for almost 30 years. A consultant on numerous National Institutes of Health grants, Knopf has served as advisor to the PBS exercise series "Sit and Be Fit," and to the State of California on disabilities issues. He is a frequent speaker at conferences and has written several textbooks and articles. Knopf is president of the Fitness Educators of Older Adults Association. He also coordinates the Fitness Therapist Program at Foothill College in Los Altos Hills, California.

acknowledgments

It is with sincere appreciation that I wish to thank the team at Ulysses Press, for without their skill and vision this book would not have been possible. People like me need people like Lily Chou and Claire Chun, whose attention to detail made my concepts become a reality. Much appreciation goes to Ashley Chase for believing in me to make this book happen. A giant thank you goes to Robert Holmes, whose ability to capture the essence of the exercises through pictures is without parallel. Lastly, thank you to the models: Toni Silver, Grant Bennett, Phyllis Ritchie, Vivian Gunderson and Mike O'Meara—they were willing to hold poses for long periods of time and exercise non-stop for several hours.